I0026910

TESTIMONIALS

"Finding the right therapist for you can be a challenge—but meeting that challenge is every bit as important as the therapy to follow. In Linda Tucker, an insightful and talented therapist, you'll find a knowledgeable guide who can stand with you at the intersections, help you read the signs and keep you on the road to success.

"Reading *At a Crossroads* is like talking to a friend who has been there before you and tells you all about it. It strikes a tone both intimate and pragmatic—the very qualities that makes therapy work. In this book, Dr. Tucker will do more than deliver answers. She will teach you and encourage you to ask questions—the right ones—that will help you get where you need to be."

MAUREEN MURPHY, PHD
FOUNDING PRESIDENT, PSYCHOANALYTIC
INSTITUTE OF NORTHERN CALIFORNIA

"This new book by Linda Tucker is a marvelous guide to the complicated path one must traverse to find a good psychotherapist. The author avoids the potholes and dead ends that are all too common in the pursuit of the therapist who is just right for you.

"I have known Linda Tucker for years, and she is a person of high integrity and uncommon wisdom. I have learned a lot from her over the years, and you will too as you absorb what she has to say in this superb volume. She manages to convey the intricacies of finding the best therapist for your needs without sacrificing the complexity of the process. I highly recommend that anyone who is contemplating therapy make this book their first stop."

GLEN O. GABBARD, MD
CLINICAL PROFESSOR OF PSYCHIATRY,
BAYLOR COLLEGE OF MEDICINE

At A Crossroads, Finding the Right Psychotherapist
Copyright ©2017 Linda Tucker

ISBN 978-1506-908-07-6 AMZ
ISBN 978-1506-904-32-0 PRINT
ISBN 978-1506-904-33-7 EBOOK

LCCN 2017942004

May 2017

Published and Distributed by
First Edition Design Publishing, Inc.
P.O. Box 20217, Sarasota, FL 34276-3217
www.firsteditiondesignpublishing.com

ALL RIGHTS RESERVED. No part of this book publication may be reproduced, stored in a retrieval system, or transmitted in any form or by any means — electronic, mechanical, photo-copy, recording, or any other — except brief quotation in reviews, without the prior permission of the author or publisher.

Library of Congress Cataloging-in-Publication Data
Tucker, Linda
    At A Crossroads, Finding the Right Psychotherapist / written by Linda Tucker.
    p. cm.
    ISBN 978-1506-904-32-0 pbk, 978-1506-904-33-7 digital

1. PSYCHOLOGY / Psychotherapy / Counseling. 2. / General. 3. /Reference.

A861

AT A CROSSROADS

Finding the Right Psychotherapist
(Even If You Already Have One)

AT A CROSSROADS

Finding the Right Psychotherapist
(Even If You Already Have One)

Linda Tucker, PsyD, LCSW

At A Crossroads: Finding the Right Psychotherapist
(Even If You Already Have One)
© 2017 Linda Tucker, PsyD, LCSW

All rights reserved under all copyright conventions. No part of this publication may be reproduced, distributed, or transmitted in any form or by any means, including photocopying, recording, or other electronic or mechanical methods, without the prior written permission of the author, except in the case of brief quotations embodied in critical reviews and certain other noncommercial uses permitted by copyright law. The scanning, uploading, and distribution of this book via the Internet or via any other means without the permission of the publisher is illegal and punishable by law. Please purchase only authorized electronic editions and do not participate in or encourage electronic piracy of copyrightable materials. Your support of the author's rights is appreciated.

This book is provided for informational purposes only and is not meant to be used, nor should it be used, to diagnose or treat any medical condition. For diagnosis or treatment of any medical problem, consult your own physician. The publisher and author are not responsible for any specific health needs that may require medical supervision and are not liable for any damages or negative consequences from any treatment, action, application or preparation, to any person reading or following the information in this book.

The use of this book does not imply nor establish any type of doctor/patient relationship and no diagnosis or treatment is being provided. The use of this book does not constitute nor offer any specific medical or psychological advice whatsoever to anyone and is not intended for that use. References are provided for informational purposes only and do not constitute endorsement of any websites or other sources. Readers should be aware that the websites listed in this book might change.

The author is not responsible for any misinterpretation of the information provided within this book or any consequences resulting from the use of these materials. The author takes no responsibility for any websites that may be linked to this book, nor implies any relationships or endorsements to any linked website.

There are those who are here to mentor us,
teach us, and give us a hand up.
This book is dedicated to the mentors and psychologists in my life
who have done that and more.

CONTENTS

Contents

FOREWORD

One of the most common concerns when people feel the need to get help from a therapist is the fear that they won't find one who is actually helpful. A secondary feeling, when one is a seeing a therapist, is often this, "Am I actually seeing the right one for me?"

Here's good news you can use. This pithy book, by a seasoned and respected psychotherapist/psychoanalyst, enables you to quell these concerns by providing a step-by-step approach, with actionable insights so you can get the best help for your psyche and situation. Her bravely candid, personal story of her path to becoming a therapist pulled me into reading the rest of this book and recommending it to others. This "coaches' coach" with 35 years of experience helping couples, individuals and nonprofit leaders enjoy more fulfilling lives, can help you too.

Use this book as a gateway to a happier, more meaningful life with others. As you can see, simply from reading the concrete chapter titles, Dr. Tucker is committed to enabling others to get the kind of *helpful* help she received—and has been providing to others, for years as a sought-after therapist.

As a long-time journalist, I am used to interviewing others. I had a life-changing experience being interviewed by Tucker for her podcast and experiencing the depth of her intuition, caring and capacity to provide concrete feedback. That experience morphed into a flourishing friendship that continues to enhance my life. I deeply believe her insights can enable you to get the therapeutic help you need so you can turn the page to the next chapter of your life adventure you were truly meant to live. And be sure to also get the free report she offers at the end: *7 Tips to Moving Forward Faster in 7 Days: How to Challenge Your Thinking and Accelerate Your Healing in Just One Week.*

                                                   –Kare Anderson

Kare Anderson is an Emmy-winning former NBC and Wall Street Journal reporter, *now connective behavior speaker and columnist for* Forbes *and* Huffington Post. *Anderson's TED talk* on The Web of Humanity: Be an Opportunity Maker *has attracted over two million views. Her clients are as diverse as Salesforce, Novartis, and The Skoll Foundation. She is the author of* Mutuality Matters, Moving From Me to We, Getting What You Want, *and* Resolving Conflict Sooner. *As David Rockefeller Jr. said after hearing her speak,* "Kare *forever changes how you see yourself and your world." Discover more at her blog* Moving From Me To We.

INTRODUCTION

I coulda been...what do you call it, Lin...a psychiatrist?" My father pronounces it *sigh-kai-uh-tryst*. "I *know* people," he continues, "always have."

I'm 35 years old and visiting my East Coast parents in the house and small town where I grew up. I moved to Manhattan and then California because I couldn't get far enough away from them. I didn't hate them; I just didn't want to become them. And I was afraid that if I stayed too long, that's exactly what would happen.

When I initially applied to college at 18 years of age, my father said, "You just don't want to work!" In other words, he had no idea what it meant to go to college. Many years later, when I was about to leave for graduate school, he offered more of his sage advice: "When are you going to get a real job?" All I could respond with was, "Are you kidding me?" and, under my breath, "What an a**hole." He couldn't hear me—and it wasn't only that he was practically deaf (literally and figuratively).

Don't get me wrong, my father offered me several things for which I am deeply grateful. He was smart as a whip, and had a work ethic that propelled him forward towards success even without a high school education. He could work circles around anyone else I have ever known then or since, and he had a sense of humor that was as quick as lightning. Unfortunately, this attribute was a double-edged sword. When you happened to be the one he was making fun of, it would strike like lightning, too.

Home was rarely a place of solace for me unless it had to do with some of my father's many sisters, particularly my Aunt Myra. She was my champion and liberator in this family. I looked forward to spending weekends with her away from the strife and sadness. I lived with an emotionally abusive older brother and bully (who accumulated seven DUI's before he lost his license for life). Amazingly, he never injured anyone with his careless driving, but he has emotionally hurt many people, including himself.

My parents really didn't like each other. They both had suffered enormous emotional losses and trauma in their childhoods. My maternal grandmother moved to New York City to become a model, leaving her three children to fend for themselves. My mother (the youngest) was three when my grandfather, overwhelmed with fear of this enormous responsibility, and heartache that his wife had abandoned him with three children, gave her up to the foster care system. Not a hopeful beginning for a toddler.

My father (the youngest of nine children) was raised during the Depression with little support and even less to eat. My paternal grandfather was both cruel and at times, loving. He owned a vegetable store on the main street in a small town and would drag his young boys out of bed at 3:00 am (before school) to go to market, where they were expected to help him load the truck.

He would open his wallet, fan the bills at his sons, and say, "You see this, boys… this is your only friend in life. Don't forget it."

What with eight siblings preceding him, by the time my father was born, his sweet and loving mother was exhausted. When I came along, many years later, the loss of the family members he loved from one malady after another left him feeling bereft. Overwhelmed by anger, disappointment and sadness (which he had no idea how to understand or to deal with constructively), he turned to alcohol and to women (other than my mother) for solace. He also began to voice what would become his favorite refrain: "I don't give a good goddamn."

My mother had two common sayings. One was for my brother: "If you don't knock it off, I'm gonna end up in Hope Dell" (the nearest mental health facility and a locked-down, scary place). The other was for me: "Thank God for you, Lin…. I would be in Hope Dell if it wasn't for you." Those words were powerful for a child to hear. In hindsight, she was probably the primary reason I became a social worker and ultimately, a psychoanalyst. I think of my mother as my first patient. She was also someone who knew the value of a good education. She encouraged my excelling in school, which became my solace.

Many children who come from difficult backgrounds turn to books, school, and teachers for a sense of comfort, safety, and sanity. Fortunately, many teachers encouraged my thinking and academic success. My mother also encouraged me to seek a spiritual life. In the beginning she forced me to go to Sunday school and church when no one else in my family had to go. I resented it at first, but now I believe that she wanted something more for me than she had been able to achieve for herself. My faith has seen me through many difficult times when I felt blindsided by what was going on at home. School and church gave me places to turn when it felt my family was failing me, and for that I feel fortunate. I have found that people who come to see me with faith—in themselves or something greater than themselves—often have an ability (or maybe it's the faith) to get better faster.

My turbulent childhood left its marks. In spite of doing well at school, in spite of being the first person in my immediate family to graduate from high school or college, and in spite of promptly moving to Manhattan, where I excelled professionally, I never felt any measurable sense of self-esteem. I didn't know what was wrong; I just knew that every day I felt sad, traumatized (I would have said depressed back then), miserable, angry, and misunderstood. The negative influences from my childhood continued to thwart the reality of my accomplishments. Nothing I did felt good enough. It was next, next, next.

Unfortunately, like most families and family members who suffer from malignant childhood environments, I had no idea what to do or to whom to turn for help. I was raised to believe that you were crazy if you went to a therapist. Even in the "Big Apple," where it seemed everyone had a "shrink," I had trouble finding someone to help me deal with my negative feelings and lack of self-worth. I saw so many therapists in my search for one with a good heart and a good mind that writing a guide of who *not* to see would have been easier than the subject of this book. My first aborted search began with a woman who directed me to talk to a pillow and to "get it all out." *Are you kidding me?* I thought. *I am not paying you to talk to a pillow.* I began to think that these therapists were crazier than I was beginning to feel in my search for someone to help me.

Trying to find a therapist when you feel so low down is difficult if not impossible. It takes courage to ask for help when you can barely get out of bed in the morning, and each time you try and fail, you become more and more discouraged. So I started to believe that no one could help me, and that it was my fault. Serendipitously, a friend casually mentioned she was going to a place called the New York Psychoanalytic Institute to talk to a therapist. She suggested that perhaps he'd see me too. (Caveat: this "share" worked back then because we were young, but it's really important to have a psychotherapist that is there for you, and one you don't have to share with a friend.)

At first I was afraid to get my hopes up again. I noticed, however, that my friend was making positive changes and progress in her life. She ended a destructive relationship and then began to take better care of herself and to make better decisions. I felt hopeful that perhaps I could be helped to change too. She gave me the name of her therapist, and with some trepidation I made an appointment.

Very quickly I discovered the difference between this doctor and other therapists I had seen. From our first session he asked probing questions—gently—that challenged my thinking. Yes, you want an empathetic and kind-hearted therapist, one you respect and feel comfortable (but not *too* comfortable) about revealing secrets you don't yet know are there. But you also want a therapist who doesn't always accept your perspective, who won't buy into your story. A good therapist must challenge your version of the narrative, and then, step by step, lead you to discover the underlying truth of your actions and life.

Within that first year of treatment, I felt I could breathe more deeply again. I had what felt like an astute collaborator guiding me towards good mental health. We worked together for three years, and then, at age 28, I moved to San Francisco, where I continued my quest for self-acceptance and knowledge with a mature, wise, and well-known woman referred by the New York Psychoanalytic Institute.

By 1992 I had spent almost fifteen years doing volunteer work concurrently with my own psychotherapy. My therapist kept asking me why I wasn't considering graduate school to become a therapist myself. I remember her telling me, "You already are 70% of the therapist you will become by the time you go to graduate school." She went on to say, "You've got what it takes. When are you going to believe that you can do what you love and get paid for it?" The truth is that I have always had a social worker's mindset. I have always given more than I got, and getting paid to do what I loved just didn't seem possible, or even kosher.

With the support and a nudge from my psychotherapist, I ultimately made the decision to become a therapist myself. However, I would not have had the courage without her foresight and belief in me. (This is the mark of a great therapist: someone who sees something in you that you don't see yourself.) I received my Master's degree in Social Work from the University of California in Berkeley, and then received post-master's training at The Psychotherapy Institute and my Doctorate in Psychoanalysis from the Psychoanalytic Institute of Northern California.

So here I am today, fortunate to work with men and women from different parts of the world from my downtown office in San Francisco. There, I help people clarify the roadblocks that prevent them from living a healthy and productive life. I love what I do, but because I lived the difficult process of finding my own therapist I decided to write this book to short-circuit that route for others. Hopefully, that includes someone like you.

When you finally find the courage to admit that you can't do it alone, you deserve support in finding the right therapist to confront your specific issues, whatever they are. You need to find someone open, trustworthy, well trained, and one who truly listens without prejudging; someone who specializes in your specific issues, and whose fees fit within your financial constraints. The journey back to health is demanding and complex and rewarding. Luckily, there are ways to shorten your search to locate, interview, and finally to select a therapist that provides a safe "holding environment"—one that facilitates looking deeply inside for the authentic you.

My hope is that this book will lighten the burden of doing just that. I sincerely wish you well.

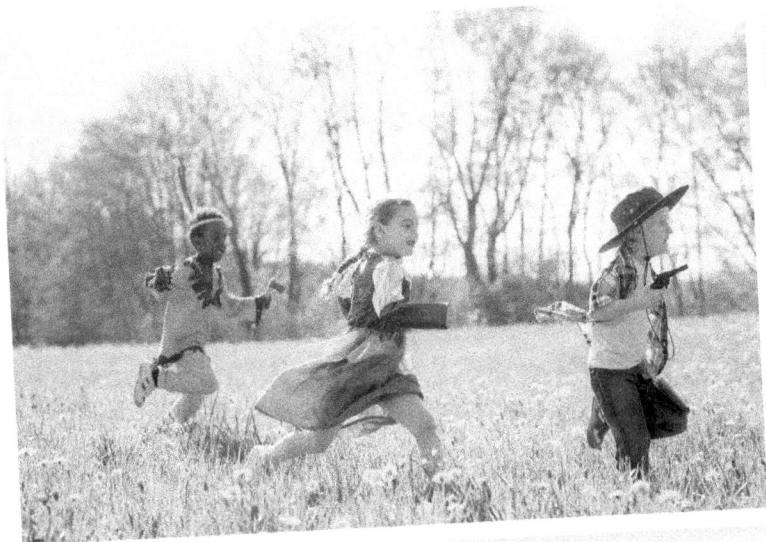

We all have that child inside of us that still needs care.

1

"WHAT'S WRONG WITH ME?"

"Desperation is sometimes as powerful
an inspirer as genius."

BENJAMIN DISRAELI

Have you ever asked yourself, "What's wrong with me?" Or asked some variation on that theme, such as, "Why don't I feel the way I used to feel?" about yourself, or someone in your life? Are you asking this question now?

Perhaps that's the reason you've opened the pages of this book. You feel something is not right with you or that your life is off-track, and you are not sure what to do about it or how to change it. Or maybe you are experiencing one (or a few) of these situations:

- You're having trouble coping with a life event such as a divorce, a death in the family, a serious illness, job loss, challenges at school, or financial difficulties.

- You've experienced a trauma or a tumultuous event and you can't seem to snap back to the way you were.

- You are unable to deal with feelings of anger, fear, or stress that, at times, overwhelm you.

- You're stuck, blocked, or aren't even sure what it is that's disturbing you. You are unable to move forward and can't figure out why.

- You might be in a relationship that is destructive and you know it, but you can't find the wherewithal to leave.

- Perhaps you are successful in your job and yet feel like a failure, or even a fraud. (You are not alone; many women especially experience this dynamic.)

- It may even be difficult for you to get out of bed, and at times you wonder why you bother to go to work. You fail to take care of yourself in the most basic ways.

- You may use food, alcohol, drugs, or excessive exercise to try to cope with difficult emotions.

- Maybe the thought has crossed your mind that it might even be better if you weren't here at all....

Whatever the reason, there is some inner voice that whispers that things aren't the way they should be; certainly not the way you want them to be. And you want—no, you need—for them to change.

I congratulate you on your motivation to consider facing the unknown, unspoken, buried truth. It's not easy to look at our lives and to realize we are unhappy. This is true especially in a culture of superlatives and superficial niceties like "have a good day," and where other's accomplishments are posted daily on Facebook and Twitter. It takes courage to admit, not only to yourself but also to someone else, that your life is far from perfect. It takes courage to admit that you can't do it alone and that you need help to change, to eliminate destructive behavior, to dump unhealthy relationships, or just to get out of bed each day.

As simplistic as it may seem, the awareness of feeling that something is wrong is a tough but essential step in the process of self-discovery and change. I encourage you to look at this moment as if you are standing at a crossroads. If you continue along the same path you've been traveling, nothing will change; indeed, your life may even get worse—more suffering, more bad choices, and more unbearable emotions.

There is, however, another option, or more appropriate, another opportunity. A crisis can be seen as an opportunity for change.

What if you could choose a new and different path instead... a path that requires you to challenge the beliefs you have held onto for such a long time?

Choosing a different path takes audacity, because it means confronting feelings and behaviors you have avoided knowing, perhaps for your entire life, such as sadness, disappointment, past mistakes, misdirected anger, unrecognized trauma, and negative self-esteem. But this is *not* a path that you have to walk without support. Help *is* available, no matter what your issue or history. You might be surprised to learn of others (friends, relatives, colleagues) who have walked this same path, gaining insight that led them to more productive and significant lives.

The first step requires a decision on your part to seek the help of a psychotherapist—someone who asks inquiring questions that point you in the direction of wholeness and away from the road of despair. Maybe this sounds too good to be true; however, finding the right psychotherapist can make it so.

Why Psychotherapy?

These days therapy is only one of many choices people make when dealing with painful emotional issues. Perhaps when you first admitted that you were unhappy you thought you could handle things on your own. When that didn't work, you may have turned to friends, family, or colleagues, who offered solutions that also didn't work. Perhaps these well-meaning people told you to "hang in there," "buck up" or "things will get better in time." Possibly things improved for a while, or remained the same. More than likely, however, they worsened.

Like me, perhaps you read a few self-help books, or attended seminars on grief, depression, trauma, PTSD, or fear of success (whatever your particular struggle), and found the advice encouraging but ultimately not helpful enough. Maybe you tried natural healing, acupuncture, meditation, herbs, diets, or exercise, but still you felt like you were bandaging a wound but ignoring the infection.

Did you visit a physician who prescribed an antidepressant or anti-anxiety medication, or any one of the dozens of drugs that are known to flatten your emotions in order to help you cope better with your world? In most cases such medications treat only the surface symptoms but not the deep, abiding causes. And while the drugs may have helped you feel a bit better, on some level you knew they weren't a long-term solution.

Unless you uncover and address the cognitive distress and the emotional cause of your unhappiness, these issues will most likely crop up again and again and produce the same unhealthy reactions and unproductive results.

Let me be clear: I am the last person to negate the value of friends, family, medication, exercise, mentors, or even self-help information, for I have benefited from all of them at different times in my life. For example, long before I became a psychotherapist I had difficulty understanding and resolving my conflicted feelings surrounding my father's death. (There were a few times when I would have liked to kill him myself—and yes, many of us have those "fantasies.") I was what I call "passively suicidal." I had no conscious desire to kill myself, but if a truck had happened to hit me while standing on the corner, I wouldn't have objected. I took antidepressants for six months to get past the worst of it, and they helped improve the nastiest of my symptoms. I realize, however, that what was most beneficial was finding and beginning to engage with a good psychotherapist. And I continue to hold that psychotherapy is the best means for handling the emotional upheavals that life serves up to all of us. I see and hear the same from colleagues who are also invested in healthy, happy and successful outcomes for their patients.

I decided to write this book because I know from my own experience that the task of finding the best psychotherapist is challenging. I believe that when you are brave enough to acknowledge the need for help—most likely at a time when you are at your wits' end—there should be a place to go for a helping hand. You deserve support to ease the way to finding the right therapist to help you pursue the path to mental health, life satisfaction, and "finding your bliss." [1]

Choosing the *Right* Therapist

I have found that therapy succeeds or falters based upon the relationship between the patient and the therapist. The good therapeutic relationship is based upon a combination of mutual trust, openness, and a willingness to speak the unspoken and the unknown truths in a benign, holding environment. (Donald Winnicott, one of my favorite psychoanalysts, coined the term "holding environment," to illustrate the optimal environment for the developing infant, one that provides the child with the security to survive the typical failures of the child-mother relationship. For me, the therapeutic relationship should replicate this concept.[2]) Above all, the relationship must be founded on compassionate caring and a commitment by the therapist to always uphold the best interests of the patient. (Note: I will use the terms "psychotherapist" and "therapist" interchangeably throughout this book.)

The relationship between therapist and patient is much like any other sustaining relationship: you feel an inexplicable rapport with some people (and some therapeutic approaches) and not with others (no talking to pillows). You need to find both the therapist and the type of therapeutic treatment that will provide the trust, rapport, and holding environment that will encourage and facilitate the best road to your mental health.

I believe the number one quality you should look for in a good therapist is that they will not only be a person who supports you, but they will also be a person who is capable of challenging your thinking in a secure, ethical environment.

For more than 20-plus years, I have worked with people to clarify whatever keeps them stuck or struggling, and eventually to uncover the causes so they may reach goals that had previously eluded them. Before I could become a person capable of guiding patients on their difficult journey, I had to "walk the walk" myself. I believe that a good therapist must undergo a deep and probing psychotherapy of his or her own. The minimal therapy hours required in most graduate schools are inadequate to steel the therapist for the emotional storms they will encounter with the patients they treat.

So, the best psychotherapists are those who have completed many years of their own psychotherapy. They are empathetic, compassionate, caring, and above all else, emotionally stable. At the same time, it is not the therapist's job to reassure you, or "kiss the boo-boo and make it all better," but to help get to the root of what is causing the anguish, the anxiety, the depression. Good therapists don't necessarily accept your explanations of why you are the way you are, or why others are always mistreating you. Instead, they persuade you to get under the surface and get clarity about your unexplored emotions, beliefs (or misbeliefs), and behaviors. They ask the tough questions and keep asking them until you recognize the authentic narrative and historical truth of your life. And they help you develop your own more mature emotions, reactions, and perspectives that encourage more evolved behavior that opens the door to psychological fitness.

I imagine by now you might be thinking, "Enough with all of this Linda…how do I find this mythic therapist, this Dr. Right?"

Most people get a referral (preferably one that their health plan approves) from their primary care doctor. (Caveat: many psychotherapists no longer accept HMO insurance because reimbursement is so miniscule. PPO insurance provides you with more options. We'll talk more about this in chapter 4.) Some ask their dentist or even their hair stylist about a therapist. Others check online rating sites. (Please be aware that some therapists who have stellar Yelp reviews are often comprised of younger and less experienced clinicians who have excellent marketing skills.)

Some search online for therapists in their community and, willy-nilly, see what websites pop up. (I caution you that it may not be the best idea because many reputable and respected therapists don't have websites. We are often an anti-tech bunch, and I am a bit of a Luddite myself. I needed a strong push to enter the 21st century and the online world. But, I digress.)

Your relationship with a psychotherapist is far more intimate than the one you have with other professionals. You don't want your doctor's Aunt Sophie's therapist (unless Aunt Sophie is rocking her world in a way you want). You *do* want someone who specializes in your specific concerns, who has rigorous training, education, and experience, and (as a secondary concern) one whose fees fit your budget. (I challenge you, however, not to be penny-wise and pound-foolish. If you believe you have found the right psychotherapist, be willing to spend the extra money.) Most importantly, you want someone with whom you will make tangible progress on those emotional hurdles.

Choosing the right psychotherapist can seem overwhelming, because when you are seeking psychological help, you are most likely not feeling at your best. You may be anxious and depressed, or in deep mourning, and as a result, feel desperate for help. Because of this, you may not be able to discern which therapist is best for you, and a Yelp review or even a recommendation from a clinic could be risky. But there are ways to shorten your search to find, interview, and select a therapist that will be the right one for you.

This book is designed to help you find a psychotherapist who will assist you in making the changes you wish to create in your life. In its pages you will find a series of questions, warnings, and ultimately, resources to help navigate the process of locating a therapist. There are many practical suggestions, as well as guidance for what to expect from this very significant therapeutic relationship. It's your precious life, and your mental health after all.

The chapters of this book cover the following:

- Some of the common reasons that people seek therapy, or should at least consider it.

- The staggering number of people who suffer from diagnosed and undiagnosed mental conditions. In other words, you are not alone.

- Choosing the right therapeutic approach for your particular challenge.

- Types of therapists and the different issues they treat.

- How to search for and locate a therapist that practices in your area. There are different resources available in larger cities than in rural areas. I will also discuss in-person versus therapy via phone or Skype.

- How to pay for therapy: there are ways to find an excellent therapist whatever your budget.

- Sources of qualified referrals, including friends and family, primary care providers, clinics, hospitals, and professional organizations. I also cover where *not* to search first. (For example, Yelp is not the best resource for this service, but it's great for others.)

- How to vet a therapist (degrees, affiliations, credentials and/or specialization, etc.), including how to check for the existence of any professional complaints.

- Making the initial contact (usually over the phone). You'll learn what to listen for and what to ask about, including schedule, fees, insurance, and all the myriad details of beginning the therapeutic relationship.

- Your first session: how comfortable are you? What can you expect? What are the warning signs that tell you that this therapist is not the one for you?

- The keys for a successful therapeutic relationship with your practitioner. You need to feel a connection and ultimately a sense of trust in order for the therapy to work.

- "Red flags" to watch out for, and how to end the ineffective therapeutic relationship.

- Clear and realistic expectations of what you will gain from therapy.

Rest assured: you can do this.

More importantly, this endeavor will be worth your effort, because the life skills you will learn, and the self- and other-understanding you will gain, will help you to live the good life you long for.

Patients frequently tell me that therapy gives them a sense of expansion. Instead of beating themselves up over past regrettable choices, they become curious about the whys and wherefores.

They become curious about their thinking and their motivation. They begin to spend more time exploring their own thinking, gaining perspective and learning to understand their feelings and past decisions. Rather than asking, "What's wrong with me?" they ask, "What can I learn from this experience? How can I move beyond my guilt and self-blame?" and, "Let me understand the decisions I've made that haven't worked out and make sure I do not repeat them. "

Many people tell me that as a result of therapy they have learned not only how to be at ease with themselves but also how to interact in healthful ways with others. Often we repeat neurotic interactions learned from our family of origin. Your relationship with your therapist can be a bridge—a paradigm, if you will— for creating improved non-neurotic relationships with partners, managers, business associates, and friends. It also can help you rid your life of toxic relationships that serve only to make you miserable. In fact, some patients report that their relationship partners and children benefit from the therapy almost as much as they have.

Others discover how to self-soothe with healthy rather than addictive activities. They develop skills to make improved choices at those moments when they are faced with tough decisions. They learn to slow down, apply their newly learned reactions to conflict, and take pride in overcoming what in the past might have led to bad choices. Most of all, they feel that they have an ally in the process. Instead of judging them for making a wrong turn, the therapist will help them explore the situation, their feelings, their projections (sometimes we attribute our own unacceptable ideas, impulses or feelings to others, and can swear it's them and not us), all of which ultimately will lead to further growth, mental health and wholeness.

After you read this book, and follow the tips it offers, it is my conviction and hope that you will feel more confident to take the leap to get the help you want and deserve. Health, hope, and life satisfaction can be yours. Take a deep breath and take the first step on this journey with me as your guide. Please turn the page and begin.

2

YOU'RE NOT ALONE: COMMON
REASONS FOR SEEKING HELP

"Life doesn't make any sense without interdependence.
We need each other, and the sooner we learn that,
the better for us all."

ERIK ERIKSON

Seeking therapy can be daunting. It takes courage to admit that we can't do it alone, and that we need help to cope with what's happening in our lives. What's worse, it can be difficult even to recognize that what we're feeling isn't typical, and that having someone tell us to "get over it," or "focus on the positive," or any of the other well-meaning things that are said by well-meaning friends and family, just doesn't work.

For many of us it's beneficial to be able to put a label on what we are feeling. For example, when you understand that the rapid breathing, feelings of suffocation, racing mind, and heart palpitations are all signs of a panic attack, you might find it easier to apply mental and physical techniques to relax, rather than thinking that you're having a heart attack, or worse, dying. Perhaps it helps to know that the anxiety and sleeplessness you experience following a particularly bad breakup or divorce are common reactions to trauma and grief.

While everyone's problems are unique, the symptoms and issues produced by those problems are often comparable and can be categorized. Modern psychotherapy is based upon our ability to assemble similar problems, symptoms, and causes together, and then to come up with a therapeutic approach that helps to restore your mental and emotional stability and well-being.

According to resources like the *Diagnostic and Statistical Manual*, 5th edition (commonly known as the *DSM–5*, it is the "bible" for psychotherapy professionals), the National Institute of Mental Health, and the National Alliance on Mental Illness, the following are the most common conditions that cause someone to seek therapy.[3]

Anxiety. This is the most prevalent mental complaint in the United States. Many people feel anxious when faced with a test, a job interview, a first date, an important meeting, or speaking to a crowd. However, an anxiety disorder is defined as *disproportionate, ongoing, and uncontrollable* worry about everyday things. An anxiety disorder can make even the most mundane of daily activities—such as going to the store, or answering the phone, or meeting someone new—an ordeal. Symptoms can include headaches, fidgeting, rapid heartbeat, sweating, nausea, irritability, fatigue, and trouble sleeping.

Depression. Symptoms include prevailing low moods, decreased self-esteem, and loss of interest in previously enjoyable activities. It is common to experience temporary feelings of depression following a significant loss, such as the death of a loved one, a job change, divorce, and so on. If such feelings are severe enough to interfere with your daily activities, or if they linger for more than two or three weeks, you should seek therapeutic help.

People who suffer from depression may also have symptoms that replicate those of an anxiety disorder, including insomnia, nervousness, irritability, and difficulty concentrating. It is common for people with anxiety disorders to also suffer from depression and vice versa. Psychotherapy helps distinguish the accurate causes of your symptoms so that you can receive appropriate treatment and relief with the right therapist.

Note: While psychiatrists (and many physicians) prescribe only antidepressants to treat depression, research demonstrates that a combination of medication and psychotherapy offers the most beneficial and long-lasting results.

Stress. Major life events such as the loss of a loved one, or a job, a car crash, a divorce, a diagnosis of a major illness—or possibly even positive life events, like childbirth, getting a promotion, or moving into a new home—typically create stress. Some people adjust to these situations quickly. Others, however, experience lingering levels of stress, and these after-effects are often debilitating.

Stress response syndrome occurs when someone develops emotional or behavioral symptoms lasting more than three months in response to a stressful situation. Physical symptoms can include heart palpitations, stomachaches, headaches, and general body aches and pains. Emotional symptoms—such as depression (hopelessness, sadness, helplessness, loss of interest in work, social withdrawal) or anxiety (nervousness, tension, impulsive behavior)—can appear as well.

While anxiety, stress, and depression are the "big three" when it comes to our mental health, there are other conditions for which people seek psychotherapy, such as:

Obsessive-compulsive disorder (OCD) is considered an anxiety disorder. People with OCD experience uncontrollable thoughts, and then they repeat actions to help decrease the anxiety produced by those thoughts. The recognition that such thoughts and behaviors are irrational further serves to increase the anxiety, which sets up a vicious cycle. Other anxiety disorders include phobias, social anxiety, hypochondria, and panic disorders.

Eating disorders include anorexia nervosa, bulimia nervosa, and binge eating disorders. All involve unhealthy and unrealistic relationships with food because of a distorted self-perception or body image. Anorexia presents as an irrational fear of gaining weight that results in extreme food restriction or exercise, or both. With bulimia, the person binges by eating an inordinate amount of food in a short amount of time, and then purges by vomiting, taking laxatives, and/or exercising excessively.

Addiction, or substance use disorders. It is possible to become addicted to different substances, behaviors, and stimulations, such as drugs (prescription and illicit), alcohol, nicotine, pornography, gambling, and the like. While some individuals can indulge in all of these activities and function fairly well, others become functionally impaired. They often exhibit loss of control, social malfunction, excessive risk taking, and other self-destructive behaviors. Ultimately, substance abuse disorders lead to health problems, and the failure to meet life's responsibilities.

With addiction, people may need to "detox" from a particular addictive substance (like alcohol, drugs, tobacco, etc.) and clear the effects of the addiction from the body. Some experts suggest that detoxification is most effective in conjunction with psychotherapy that addresses the emotional, as well as the physical, causes of addiction. Other experts suggest the need to rid the body of all toxic substance prior to starting psychotherapy. This decision will ultimately depend on the psychotherapist's training and philosophy.

Impulse control disorders. Impulse control disorder sufferers feel the urge to act in ways that could harm themselves or others. You may be familiar with some impulse control disorders such as kleptomania (uncontrollable stealing) or pyromania (the uncontrollable setting of fires). Other, less familiar versions include cutting (oneself, or objects), or hair pulling.

Post-traumatic stress disorder (PTSD). By now most people are familiar with, or have read about, veterans and/or survivors of trauma caused by war, rape, and sexual abuse that have resulted in PTSD. Individuals who experience natural disasters or who witness a serious crash may also suffer symptoms of PDSD, such as flashbacks, nightmares and hyper-vigilance.

Personality disorders. Personality disorders have names such as borderline, avoidant, antisocial, dependent, sociopathic, and narcissistic. People with personality disorders usually display extreme, inflexible, and rigid personality traits. Things are either/or, right or wrong, black or white, with no shades of gray. Such people can appear odd or eccentric, dramatic or overly emotional, difficult, or anxious and fearful. While they tend to believe that their view of the world and way of being is "right" (even though it is very different from that of others), they have very narrow limits of what is acceptable in themselves and others, and they have trouble dealing with the changes and demands of everyday life and work.

Sexuality and gender issues. This includes conflicts relating to sexual desire, performance, and/or behavior, such as challenges with arousal (or the lack of it), or sexual fantasies, urges, or behaviors that are distressing or disabling. Issues of gender identity and expression include the sense that one's emotional and psychological identity does not correspond with their assigned sex.

Suicidal thoughts. At one point or another, many people have thought about suicide. Of course, any type of suicidal thought should be a signal to seek out therapy. When suicidal thoughts become habitual, however, or if someone moves from passive thoughts (a nonspecific desire to die) to an active one (not only a wish to die but a plan to do it) then it is essential to intervene immediately. If this is you, or someone you know, please contact the suicide prevention hotline in your area NOW.

Please note that the above is only a partial list of common life complaints for which people think about seeking psychotherapy. You may or may not find your particular set of symptoms on the list, but if in the quiet of the night, your own inner voice is telling you that things are not right, trust it.

Why It's Important to Get Help: the State of Mental Health in the U.S.

As I said in the title of this chapter, you are not alone when you feel the need for help to deal with your unhappy feelings.

Millions of people in the United States suffer from diagnosed and undiagnosed mental problems ranging from mild to severe. Here are a several significant statistics about mental health in the U.S.[4]

- In 2014 approximately 43.6 million people age 18 or older in the U.S. had some form of mental illness in the previous year. This equates to more than 18% of the U.S. adult population, or *one in every 5.5 adults.*

- More than 9.8 million adults—one in every 25—experienced serious mental illness in 2014. ("Serious" is defined as any illness that substantially interferes with or limits one or more major life activities.)

- The numbers are worse for young adults: *almost half* (46.3%) of the people in the U.S. between ages 13 and 18 will experience a mental disorder at some time in their lives, and 21.4% of them will have severe mental disorders.

- According to research from 2012, more than 21% of adults (42.5 million) in the U.S. are affected by anxiety disorders each year. And fewer than 37% were receiving any kind of mental health care treatment.

- The prevalence of depression is not much better. In 2015, 6.7% of adults in the U.S., or 16.1 million people, had at least one major depressive episode in the previous 12 months.

- *46.4% of Americans will have a diagnosable mental illness in their lifetime.* The lifetime risk of major depression in adults is approximately 17%.

- In 2014 there were 20.2 million adults in the U.S. with a substance use disorder. Of that group, more than 50.5%, or 10.2 million people, had a co-occurring mental illness.

- Suicide is the 10th leading cause of death in the U.S, costing more than 41,000 lives each year. That's more than double the number of lives lost annually to homicide.

- Some estimates of the cost of mental disorders to the U.S. economy (including the cost of treatment combined with lost earnings and public disability insurance payments) were at least $467 billion in 2012.

And here, to my mind, is the most tragic statistic of all:

- **In 2014, only *41%* of adults with a mental health condition received services to treat that condition in the previous year.**

Please, don't be one of the 59% of those people with a mental health condition who suffer silently and alone, when there are ways to get proper treatment. In the next chapter, I will walk you through the process of finding a therapist to help you with whatever challenges you face. Above all, remember, you're not alone. Help is available. It will just take a little diligence on your part to locate the best therapist for you.

3

STARTING YOUR SEARCH

"Our doubts are traitors,
And make us lose the good we oft might win,
By fearing to attempt."

Lucio in Shakespeare's Measure for Measure

Now that you have made the decision to get help, the next step is to determine the *right* help for your particular condition and situation. There are two primary roads when it comes to treating psychological issues. One is the medical/medication route that I discussed in chapter 1. And, of course, medication is appropriate in some circumstances—overcoming addiction often requires medical treatment for withdrawal, for instance, or bipolar disorder can benefit from medication that balances the body's chemistry.

Psychotherapy is the second road—and it's the one that I believe can have the greatest positive impact on your challenges. Of course, as a practicing psychotherapist and psychoanalyst for 20-plus years, I am biased in favor of the positive results of therapy, but there are numerous studies and lots of data to back up my point of view. In psychotherapy, you and a psychotherapist talk through whatever is going on that brought you there. Therapy is designed to help you explore past traumas and internal obstacles and to resolve any current problems you face.

The goal of psychotherapy is for you to develop behaviors and attitudes that will increase your emotional well-being and resilience and make you feel and do better in general. Psychiatric disorders like obsessive-compulsive disorder or anxiety can respond well to different forms of psychotherapy, for instance. Even if you are currently on medication, you should consider psychotherapy as a vital means of surpassing the emotional barriers that keep you from leading a productive life with greater mental health.

NOTE: This book is for people who are interested in finding a *private practice clinician*. You may be seeking other kinds of therapy or therapists, or you may feel you need medical management of your condition. If so, while you may find some suggestions in this book helpful, other recommendations will likely not apply to you.

Which Kind of Therapist Should You Seek?

When you begin your search (and we'll talk about how to do that in the next two chapters), you may be confounded and confused by the variety of different clinicians out there. In the main, psychotherapists can be put in a few basic categories.

Psychiatrists: Medical doctors (MDs) who have done internships and residencies in psychiatry. Their expertise is in the medical diagnosis, management, and prevention of mental health disorders. Because they are also MDs, psychiatrists can prescribe medication, so typically they treat conditions such as bipolar disorder, clinical depression, and schizophrenia. Many psychiatrists use psychotherapy in conjunction with medication to treat their patients.

Psychologists: Psychologists (who hold either a PhD, PsyD, or DSW) focus on treating patients with mental and emotional issues. They focus on behavior and the thoughts, feelings and motivation underlying such behavior, and they treat patients using psychotherapy (although a few states allow psychologists to prescribe medication as well). Many psychologists specialize in a particular therapeutic approach (like cognitive-behavioral therapy, for example), but they also adapt their methods to suit the needs of the specific patient. Psychologists also do psychological testing.

Psychoanalysts: Psychoanalysis is based upon the premise that thoughts, feelings, and behavior are motivated in part by unconscious (and often unresolved) influences from our past. By bringing these thoughts and emotions to conscious awareness, and then helping the individual to clarify and understand the (at times) misunderstood meaning of their thoughts and emotions, patients feel better and are thus better able to interact with their environment and the people in it. Psychoanalysts are trained (generally for five additional years of clinical training and postgraduate work) to guide patients in this complex process, which can produce a profound transformation even when other therapies have failed.

Marriage and Family Therapists: MFTs work with individuals, couples and families (including children), to enhance the quality of relationships within the family. The focus is often on understanding the dynamics among family members and improving communication and healthy functioning within the family unit. MFTs (and psychoanalysts, for that matter) have extensive training in how the issues of each person in the family affect the others, and how the interplay between family members can cause conflicts both within and outside the home. They then work with the family as a group, and with its individual members, to understand and resolve the dynamics and prior difficulties, leading to increased psychological health.

(The somewhat confusing caveat: Psychoanalysts and psychiatrists can also provide couples and family therapy. Look for the clinician's experience and the number of years in practice. MDs, PhDs, PsyDs, and DSWs all have four-plus additional years of training and licensure than MFTs and LCSWs.)

Licensed Clinical Social Workers: When I graduated from UC Berkeley School of Social Welfare in 1992, the LCSW was one of the more rigorous licenses to get in the State of California. LCSWs receive clinical training in therapy and counseling. They may work in schools and public health settings, as well as in private practice. LCSWs offer therapy designed to focus on a patient's strengths and talents, taking into account not only the individual's psychology and emotions but also the social and environmental factors at play. Patients consult LCSWs, in particular, when emotional, and behavioral issues affect their interactions with the outside world. LCSWs also work with patients who have substance abuse and relationship difficulties.

In general, "psychotherapist" is a catchall term used to describe psychiatrists, psychologists, psychoanalysts, counselors, MFTs, LCSWs, and other mental health professionals. Because they are all required to have specialized training in psychotherapy, finding a suitable psychotherapist—whether a marriage and family therapist, social worker, psychologist, psychiatrist, or psychoanalyst—may not be the daunting task you feared.

What Kind of Therapy Might Be Best for You?

When you begin your search for the right psychotherapist, one of the questions you will need to consider is the kind of therapy that is best for your issue. There are many different approaches and schools of therapy, and one or more of them may be appropriate.

Let's talk about a few of the most common psychotherapy approaches: medical, psychodynamic, cognitive-behavioral, and interpersonal/family therapy.

Medical: Medical therapy uses medication (prescribed by a psychiatrist) to treat psychological issues with an underlying biological or neurochemical component. Consider medical therapy if you believe that you have (or have been diagnosed with) schizophrenic, clinical depression or bipolar disorder, or are addicted to a chemical substance. Ideally, however, you should consider other forms of "talk therapy," as most people with psychological issues do better when they receive psychotherapy as part of their treatment.

Psychodynamic: An explorative therapy approach designed to go more deeply into the unconscious (unknown to you in the moment) influences and past history. Moreover, it examines past and present thoughts and feelings in greater depth. The psychotherapist will encourage you to talk freely about your thoughts (whatever comes to mind in any given moment), feelings and memories, and will help you uncover how the past affected your present problems leading to healthier choices.

Psychoanalysis is the gold standard of psychodynamic therapy. As I previously mentioned, psychoanalysts have five-plus years of additional/required clinical training. Because this process plumbs the depth of the psyche and uncovers previously unknown barriers to healthy behavior, it often takes longer than other forms of psychotherapy. (One way to think about it is that it took years to get to this place of discomfort, and it will likely take more time to get out of it.) To facilitate the psychoanalytic treatment, you will be seen multiple times per week.

Some psychotherapists and even psychoanalysts (depending on your condition) offer short-term psychodynamic therapy, which unfolds over the course of 20 sessions.

Consider psychodynamic therapy (usually offered by psychoanalysts or psychoanalytically-trained psychotherapists) if your goal is to get at the roots of conscious and unconscious patterns of thinking, feeling, and acting, to resolve past traumas, and to rid yourself of the internal obstacles that previously blocked your path to wellbeing and success.

Cognitive behavioral therapy (CBT): In CBT, the therapist encourages you to explore and recognize the impact of your present thought processes or behaviors, and identify any dysfunctional patterns that contribute to the obstacles you face. Once such patterns are identified, with the assistance of the therapist you work to change the thought patterns that have negatively influenced your moods or actions. From that perspective, you work to develop and practice strategies to modify the unwanted behaviors.

CBT is usually structured; it is shorter in duration than psychodynamic therapy because it focuses primarily on current problems and often does not delve into the past or the reasons underpinning your present situation.

Consider CBT if you have certain habitual, unwanted behavioral and thought patterns. CBT therapists concentrate on conditions such as obsessive-compulsive disorders, anxiety disorders, and social phobias. Some addiction patterns (smoking cessation, for instance) also benefit from CBT.

Interpersonal/family therapy: This method of treatment focuses on the vicissitudes of your relationships with others, and looks for patterns that create conflict and distress. The emphasis is less upon your thoughts and feelings and more upon dysfunctions in your interactions with others. When you learn better interpersonal skills, healing is possible and your reward will be greater happiness, enhanced self-esteem and confidence. Interpersonal/family therapy often includes other people (a spouse, children, parents, and so on), as successful treatment requires change in all members of the relationship.

Consider interpersonal/couples/family therapy if your issues primarily arise when you are dealing with difficulties in your relationships.

There are many different forms of therapy that fall into these four categories. Group therapy, for example, can be psychodynamic, CBT, or interpersonal in practice, depending upon the issues being addressed. You may find group therapy most beneficial if, under the guidance of a trained group counselor, you find it helpful to listen, share and exchange perspectives with others facing similar challenges. Art therapy, play therapy for children, integrative therapy, spiritual psychology—all use elements of the four categories to foster change.

Two Key Questions to Consider

To determine the best kind of therapy and therapist, first ask yourself, *"What kind of change do I want?"* Do you have a behavior you want to modify or eliminate? A way of responding to the world that no longer works (or perhaps never worked)? Do you have a problem primarily with your relationship with your spouse, children, parents, or siblings, or your colleagues/boss at work? Do you want to get rid of anxiety, a phobia, depression, underlying anger, or a sense of alienation from others and the world?

Perhaps you are not quite sure of what you want to change, only that you know that what you're doing and experiencing now isn't the way you want to live your life. Then you would be best served by asking, *"What kind of therapy feels right for me?"* Is this something you want to handle (or at least try to handle) with cognitive therapy? Do you feel more comfortable looking at yourself in the presence of others with similar problems (group therapy)? Are you curious about what makes you tick, so that confronting your history, the unknown parts of yourself, and your inner reality by probing more deeply into the internal obstacles that have prevented you from achieving your goals using psychoanalytic psychotherapy is for you?

Again, I must admit to a bias based upon my years of experience seeing patients in psychoanalytic psychotherapy and psychoanalysis and, as I've mentioned, these two kinds of therapy, in particular, changed my life. I believe too many people (or their doctors) use medication as the only remedy. They try to medicate their feelings away rather than doing the challenging and scary labor of facing their feelings and making the changes that will ultimately ameliorate the anxiety or depression. Medication can be a valid short-term solution, or a long-term option when used to address a chemical imbalance. Medication used for a prolonged period, however, can be problematic. If you choose medication, please be certain to pursue additional psychotherapy to get to the bottom of the issues you may understandably fear to face. We don't become depressed for no reason. Unless you truly understand the underlying reasons for your distress, they are most likely to repeat.

I believe in short-term therapy if there is a short-term problem. However, short-term therapy can at times fail to address the essential roots of the issue. If you are dealing with something specific in your life—a short but painful transition, a stubbornly resistant behavior for instance—then seeing a psychotherapist for brief therapy for a specific reason might be perfectly adequate. If, however, something's been plaguing you for a long time, or if you're doing well in most areas of your life but you are still stuck in other areas, or if you are excellent at figuring things out for other people but not so good at your own stumbling blocks, then therapy that addresses the roots of your problems may be the way to go. If you don't get beneath the top layer of your distress to see the underside, you will not resolve it. My advice is to find a therapist who can help you dig deep.

Here is the key: If you try one kind of therapy and things are good for a while and then the issue recurs, it hasn't been resolved. You may then want to re-consider and commit to a more thorough, in depth treatment: psychoanalytic psychotherapy or psychoanalysis.

REMINDER AND WARNING: If you are having suicidal thoughts or contemplating suicide, please seek help immediately. Most communities have suicide hotlines, or you should inform your medical doctor so he or she can get you the help you need ASAP.

In the next chapter I will talk about some of the practical concerns of finding a psychotherapist in your area, and paying for your treatment.

4

PRACTICAL CONCERNS: FINDING THERAPY WHERE YOU LIVE, AND HOW TO PAY FOR IT

"A wise person should have money in their head,
but not in their heart."

JONATHAN SWIFT

When you search for a psychotherapist, it's wise to consider a number of practical things. In this chapter I will discuss the best way to find a therapist where you live, and how to pay for it.

Where Do You Live?

If you are in or near an urban area, you have more options when it comes to psychotherapists. In a more rural community, the number of practitioners available may be smaller, and they may or may not specialize in your particular problem. Certainly, these practitioners may provide excellent treatment; you simply want to make sure that *whatever* therapist you choose is a match for your needs in terms of personality, expertise, and therapeutic approach.

If you wish a greater selection of therapists, or if you feel that the local practitioners don't meet your needs, or perhaps if you're concerned about confidentiality in your small community, there is another option. Many practitioners now offer therapy sessions via phone and/or Skype, which makes it possible to find one with the expertise and character you require who will work with you long-distance.

Phone or Skype therapy has both advantages and disadvantages. For example, on the pro side, therapy via phone or Skype with a clinician who doesn't live in your community may help preserve your anonymity. Such a therapist may be more objective because they are not influenced by local politics or personalities. Therapists from smaller towns are likely to know most everyone and may not be able to be as objective as needed. On the con side, therapists from a different geographic area might not know the culture and dynamics of the local community, and they might miss something that a local therapist would notice and address. (Always make sure that the therapist you seek via phone or Skype is licensed to provide long distance therapy.)

While many therapists who offer sessions via phone or Skype are good at reading tone of voice and body language, even at a distance, there is something powerful about face-to-face therapy. Sitting in the same room with patients and feeling and seeing their reaction is an important part of the therapeutic process for me. Having the right "witness" can be a very powerful healing experience. A stronger bond develops, along with a stronger level of commitment when meeting in-person. As patients, we are less likely to cancel sessions or terminate therapy when that bond is powerful and supportive. And showing up in life and in therapy is half the battle.

(Caveat: I have conducted therapy over the phone but prefer to have an established, face-to-face connection, or at least have had an opportunity to meet the person I will be working with. I want to make sure I can help someone before I commit to working with him or her.)

Bottom line: it is possible to find a great therapist no matter where you live. I recommend that you first research clinicians close by, and then look for therapists who specialize in your particular issue who practice in cities and/or universities in your area. If you find someone more than an hour away who seems just right, simply call or email and ask if they offer sessions via phone or Skype.

Whether the therapist is local or resides in another community, be certain to go through the vetting and initial interview processes outlined in chapters 4 and 5, to determine whether he or she is right for you.

How to Pay for Therapy: Health Insurance

Many people have financial constraints to consider when it comes to paying for therapy. After all, psychotherapy usually requires multiple sessions over weeks, months, or years, and the cost can be significant. And while some therapists will adjust their rate to accommodate your budget, it remains a large financial obligation. Please note that the more experienced a clinician is, the less likely they will work on a sliding scale. It is also less likely they will be listed on any HMO panels. For more senior psychotherapists, you should expect to pay full fee and assume they will have waiting lists for treatment. Don't despair: there are still many junior but excellent and well-trained therapists from which to choose. Or, if you feel you can wait, getting on the therapist's waiting list is always a possibility.

It is likely that some mental health care coverage is included in your health insurance plan. Since 2008 federal law requires that mental health care is treated on par with physical health care. However, health care law has been known to change, and health plans may differ in what they cover. Check your "Description of Plan Benefits" to see what types of mental health services are covered, and what, if any kind of treatment, is excluded. And, be sure to read the fine print.

If you have financial constraints, start by checking the list of providers that offer psychotherapy through your insurance plan and type of coverage. A Health Maintenance Organization (HMO) will only allow you to visit certain doctors and hospitals within their network. (A network is generally made up of providers that have agreed to see patients for lower fees.) Most HMOs will have very specific lists of approved practitioners, and if you see anyone not on the list, you have to pay the full cost of treatment yourself.

A Preferred Provider Organization (PPO) will allow you to visit whatever healthcare provider you choose without having to get a referral from a primary care physician (which is what HMOs require). With a PPO plan, there may be a larger number of psychotherapists you can consult whose fees will be covered in part by your insurance. However, there is likely to be a list of "approved" mental health practitioners whose services are covered under your particular plan, and if you select someone outside of your insurer's approved list, your insurance may or may not reimburse you for the cost of treatment. Mental health coverage is subject to the same financial conditions as physical health coverage. Depending on your plan, there will be a co-payment for each session, and any out-of-pocket expenditure over that amount will be counted toward your plan's yearly deductible.

Choosing a particular therapist from a list provided by your insurer can be daunting because all the names are unfamiliar. While I don't advocate using Google to find a psychotherapist, doing an internet search on a particular therapist can provide some great initial information. Google the therapist for any online data, and make sure to see if there are any complaints filed against them.

Please note: As I mentioned earlier, many senior therapists (those who have been practicing for many years) are electing not to deal with health insurers at all. The hassle factor of billing, forms, and refusal of verifiable claims is burdensome. In these cases, the responsibility of payment is yours. But don't despair: you may still be able to submit the therapist's invoices for partial reimbursement. Check your insurance plan's guidelines to determine the precise terms of coverage. To avoid any surprises, be sure to check with your Human Relations Department or insurance provider.

How to Pay for Therapy If You Lack Insurance (or the Therapist You Want to See Is Not in Your Network)

If you lack health insurance, or your plan does not offer coverage for the treatment you seek, or if you simply can't afford the fees for long-term therapy, there are other lower-cost options available. University students, for example, can find practitioners through their campus health center. And, depending on your financial circumstances, you may be able to receive treatment at mental health clinics run by psychotherapy training institutes, hospitals, and state and local government agencies that offer low- or no-cost treatment. *Please* make sure to look for clinics with established reputations, even though they often have waiting lists. If you are not in a crisis, it is best to wait for the person or place with the best reputation.

Group therapy is another viable option that typically offers lower fees. There are groups for almost every issue, including grief counseling, alcoholism, drug addiction, sexual addiction, rape, incest, divorce, trauma, suicide, eating disorders, depression, anxiety, and the like. Often therapists that lead such groups are volunteers who work in that particular specialty to gain more experience, or because they have an interest or personal experience in the topic area. If you go to group therapy and feel a special connection to the therapist, and you feel you want one-on-one therapy, ask if he/she will accept you as a private client and what the fee would be.

Finally, graduate students, doctoral students, and post-doctoral candidates at universities or centers that train psychotherapists are often excellent sources of affordable care. These students (who are mostly therapists in training) are under the supervision of experienced therapists in their particular program and thus *more* likely to be well trained and dedicated. The bonus is that the fees for appointments with such student psychotherapists are often very affordable.

I am a big proponent of considering graduate student therapists because I was one once. When I was a graduate student at The Psychotherapy Institute, I had a full patient roster. (Believe it or not, that is one predictor of success and can and should be a determining factor to finding a good therapist. Find someone that others want to see. A popular therapist by and large will be someone worth the wait.) I believe that you can receive great treatment from well-trained therapists who are at the beginning of their careers.

How should you decide whether a particular student practitioner is right for you? Check out their supervising professor/therapist. If the supervisor has a good reputation, he/she will be likely to attract the best students. Of course, you need to see if the student therapist is a match for your needs and style, just as you would with any therapist.

Don't Be Afraid to Talk Fees

I will go through the initial conversation with a prospective therapist in chapter 5, but I want to emphasize that you should never be reluctant to ask a therapist about his or her fees during your initial contact. The therapist's fees may be beyond your financial means, so knowing that in the first session (before you establish a bond with the therapist) is so much better than finding it out later and then having to sever the relationship. In fact, to avoid a charge that is beyond your means, ask about fees during the initial phone call. Should that happen, ask the therapist for a recommendation of someone who might (1) be in your plan, (2) charge less, or (3) offer a sliding fee scale.

That said, a first-class psychotherapist who can help you get the results you want is worth a lot. Would you rather go to someone simply because they are covered by your insurance plan, or whose fees you can easily afford, but end up unhappy with your progress during therapy? Of course, there are good psychotherapists available in many insurance plans and who charge a wide range of fees. But ultimately the question is, are they the right therapist for *you*? If the therapist you select provides the help you need to jump over the hurdles you have erected (through no fault of your own), they will be worth whatever the cost. Would you take your car to someone who ultimately cannot fix it? And, if you can't afford to fix your car, how creative would you get to obtain the funds to do so? Be creative and don't be afraid to ask for help from those you know (family and otherwise).

Don't let finances be the ultimate barrier to securing the therapy and the help you require. Look at therapy as a worthwhile investment in your health and well-being. With a little research, there are ways to find an excellent therapist whatever your budget and wherever you live. That's the subject of our next chapter.

5

FINDING AND VETTING A THERAPIST

"The past is what makes the present coherent,
and the past will remain horrible for exactly as long as
we refuse to assess it honestly."

James Baldwin, Notes of a Native Son

There are four places that I believe you should use as resources for qualified referrals, and a few places you might avoid. I will describe each in order of the best-case scenario.

#1. Family and Friends

The best source for a referral to a psychotherapist is a family member or friend (assuming you have a family you can trust). Do you know someone who has been in therapy and made great strides? You know these people best and can see for yourself whether they have made progress. For example, suppose that you are having problems with your spouse, partner, or significant other, and you recall that a friend or family member, "Sam," went through a bad divorce a few years ago. Now Sam is remarried, and he seems really happy. It would be logical to ask Sam if he had counseling back then and if so, might he recommend his therapist.

If you don't know anyone that has ever been in therapy, perhaps you may have witnessed someone in your circle of friends and family who seemed to be going through a tough time and now they appear to be doing better. Don't be afraid to ask them what they did to help themselves. You may very well find that they are (or were) in therapy, and they may be willing to share the name of their therapist. Fortunately, today therapy isn't something people are reluctant to discuss. In fact, I have noticed just the opposite. People who have excellent results in therapy are often eager to talk, not only about their therapy but also about their psychotherapist. (This may be more valid in urban areas than in smaller communities—but you never know.)

Of course, you want to be smart about the friends or family members you ask for a recommendation. Are they people you trust? Do they share your values and way of life? Appraise whether they have made progress, or ask a mutual friend if they have noticed what you seem to be noticing. Family members, partners, and spouses are often the first to notice and approve of the changes they see in their loved one. At times, I have heard (through my patients) how grateful members of their families are for the transformations they've witnessed. One patient once told me, "My son wants to thank you. He says that since I've started seeing you I've stopped being an a**hole."

#2. Universities, Institutes, and Psychotherapy Training Programs

If none of your friends or family members have experienced therapy (although it's very possible they have and you simply don't know about it), the next best place to look for a referral is at universities, psychotherapy institutes, and other programs in your area that train psychotherapists. These institutions often have counseling centers where you can find a therapist, or they may have a list of therapists to whom they refer patients.

You can do a Google search on "top psychotherapy training programs," or "psychotherapy training programs," or "psychoanalytic training programs," with the name of your city included in the search term ("top psychotherapy training programs Minneapolis," for example). That should bring up a list of the programs available through universities, psychotherapy institutes, and graduate training programs in your area. (In San Francisco, where I live, the Access Institute for Psychological Services offers an excellent program for post-doctoral candidates, many of whom also see patients.) I did such a Google search recently on "top psychotherapy training programs San Francisco," and, apart from paid advertisements, these were the top results:

- San Francisco Psychoanalytic Psychotherapy Training Program

- San Francisco Center for Psychoanalysis

- Palo Alto Psychoanalytic Psychotherapy Training Program

- San Francisco Psychoanalytic Psychotherapy Training Center & Internships

- Psychoanalytic Psychotherapy Training/APsaA

On the websites of these programs you will find a list of the people with MD or PhD degrees who are on the programs' advisory boards. You can call the board members or Advisory Board Members and ask them if they have time to assist you; tell them what you need, and ask them for a referral. The chances are good that these board members themselves have worked with most diagnostic categories (or know someone who has) and would be happy to share that information. (If you find the thought of "cold calling" an institution or board member daunting, ask a more assertive friend for help.)

I believe that board and advisory board members are excellent sources of referrals for three reasons. First, psychotherapists that serve as board members usually know the best therapists in your area. They also know which therapists they are *less* likely to recommend. (More on that later in this chapter.)

Second, many of the people who teach or train students in the universities, institutes, and training programs also accept private patients. Most good psychoanalysts or psychotherapists teach or have taught in the past. Those who teach are usually affiliated with these institutions; such a therapist must stay up to date, not only on the latest research but also on the most effective therapeutic modalities. For that reason they continue to learn and to grow, which is a good thing for any therapist. As I mentioned earlier, however, these therapists often have waiting lists.

Third, if finances are a concern, the post-graduate and post-doctoral students at these universities, institutes, and training programs are excellent choices for low- or even no-cost therapy. Don't hesitate to contact the teachers or board members of any of these programs to ask which of their students they would recommend. They know which students are excelling and which to recommend for your particular situation. Board members or professors put their own reputations on the line whenever they refer people to their students, and for that reason, the referral will most likely to be to a competent psychotherapist.

Another approach is to call and ask for the counseling department of the psychotherapy training programs in your area (or see if you can get the phone number online). Then describe exactly what you are looking for—the kind of issue you wish to address, if you prefer to see a man or a woman, if you have a preference to the amount of experience the therapist has, etc. Often you will receive recommendations for therapists that fit your needs.

#3. Your Primary Care Physician

Whenever you need to consult a specialist for a physical problem, you would probably call your primary care physician (or another physician with whom you have an ongoing relationship) to ask him or her for the best referral. That is also the first step many people take when they look for a psychotherapist. I would, therefore, like to suggest a few considerations for you to ponder when you ask your family doctor for a recommendation.

First, unless your primary care physician refers regularly to a therapist (and your doctor has been pleased with the results of past referrals), chances are he will simply consult the list of therapists available through a local hospital or clinic, and choose someone at random. If your physician recommends a therapist, it's vital that you know (1) the last time your doctor recommended the therapist (was it several years ago or last month?), and (2) the results of that treatment (of course without releasing any confidential information).

Second, when one raises certain psychological issues (like depression or anxiety) to a primary care physician, it's possible that the doctor will suggest you first try medication and then pursue therapy. But remember: according to research, medication is often more effective when taken in conjunction with psychotherapy. In this case, asking for a referral to a psychiatrist (who can prescribe medication) may be the best approach.

If you do ask your primary care physician for a referral to a psychotherapist, make sure you ask the following questions:

- How did you hear about this therapist?

- Have you referred other patients to this therapist?

- Do you regularly refer people to him/her?

- How many years have you been sending people to this therapist?

- What did those patients say about the therapist and the therapy?

- How long did those patients see the therapist?

- Did the therapy help?

Most doctors are trained to be helpful to their patients and to guide them to specialists when necessary, so it makes sense that should you request a referral from your primary care physician, he or she will want to provide you with a name. Please remember it is your responsibility to make sure that the referral will be the best therapist for your particular situation.

#4. Clinics, Hospitals, and Professional Organizations

Depending on where you live, local clinics, community health centers, and hospitals may provide referrals for psychological services. You can check the clinic or hospital directory for a social worker or therapist specializing in your particular issue. Even if you don't want to go to a clinic or hospital, they can provide you with a list of referrals.

Your church, synagogue, mosque or member of the clergy also can be a good source for referrals. If you are a college or university student, check out the campus health center, as most universities today offer mental health counseling. Sometimes larger companies have mental health referral services for employees as well. You can check your list of employee benefits, or contact your Human Resources Department to see what's available (and what may be covered as part of your health insurance). Some people prefer that their employers not know they are seeking therapy. If that is your concern, there are other excellent referral resources available, as I have previously described.

Where *Not* to Go

It used to be that if you were looking for a doctor, attorney, accountant, or other such professional, you turned to a trusted business colleague or a friend to suggest someone they consulted. While people may resort to that, it's now more common to seek referrals on the internet. After all, we Google people we want to date; we Google potential business associates or hair stylists or exercise studios or plumbers or other service providers. Why not search for a therapist online?

Two reasons. First, many of the most experienced and talented therapists don't even have an online site. I kid you not. Only in the past few years has it become customary for professionals, such as attorneys, accountants, and medical doctors to use websites to advertise their services. (In fact, at one time, it was against the law for doctors and psychologists to advertise at all.) Many experienced psychotherapists are behind the curve when it comes to listing themselves online in anything other than a more discreet professional directory.

Second, the therapists who *do* have an online site and get themselves listed "number one" on a Google search may be very good at keywords and search engine optimization (SEO), but not as good as psychotherapists. The internet, for some, remains a little like the "Wild West" when it comes to listing psychotherapists. And unfortunately, many people, including therapists, make unfounded promises or represent themselves and their results in the most laudatory, but misleading way, without proof of performance.

You *can* use Google or other search engines to look for psychotherapy training programs in your area, or to find clinics that specialize in your particular issue, but locating a program or a clinic is only the first step. From there, you need to call or email to get their recommendations for therapists to contact.

Other places you may want to avoid when looking for a therapist:

- If you want a burrito, window washer, plumber, restaurant recommendation or the like, Yelp can help—but it's unlikely to do so when you want a qualified referral to an excellent therapist.

- Stay away from the Yellow Pages, White Pages or any other directory where practitioners can be listed for free or for a low fee. There is no oversight for these listings, and half of them list you whether you have submitted any information about yourself anyway. You need to know where a referral comes from, and a listing in a directory does not guarantee expertise or experience.

Once you have a valid recommendation from a qualified source, please *do* look up the therapist online as a background check. Therapists associated with a particular clinic, hospital, organization or institute may have their biography listed on the organization's website. If you do find a web page that lists a therapist you find interesting, see what information is provided on that page about the therapist's credentials, including their training, current professional affiliations, and where they practice.

Checking a Therapist's Credentials

Once you have a referral for a psychotherapist, your next step is to check the practitioner's credentials: where they studied, where they received their degrees, where they have practiced, their specializations in particular types of therapy, and so on. Usually you can find this information through the various licensing and professional boards in your state. In California, for example, you can go on the website for the California Board of Psychology, or the Board of Behavioral Sciences, type in the name of a therapist, and verify that this person is licensed to practice in the state.

Above all else, please make sure there have been no complaints filed about this therapist, or that there are no disciplinary actions by the state or professional boards. Complaints that are filed with a state board or the American Psychological Association usually go through a process to verify the incident and then, if warranted, to take suitable disciplinary action. Although it is possible for a good therapist to be the subject of an unfounded complaint by an unhappy patient, a disciplinary action indicates that the psychology board or board of behavioral sciences validated that complaint. If you are considering a therapist with multiple complaints or a disciplinary action listed on the record, I hope you will seriously reconsider that decision.

Once you have completed the background search and feel satisfied with your choice and his or her bona fides, your next step is to speak directly with the therapist. Take a deep breath, pick up the phone, and make the call. I cover the initial phone call in the following chapter.

6

THE INITIAL CALL AND
FIRST APPOINTMENT

*"Don't ask what the world needs. Ask what makes you come
alive, and go do it. Because what the world needs
is people who have come alive!"*

HOWARD WASHINGTON THURMAN

Congratulations—hopefully, you have narrowed your list of potential therapists to one, or maybe two. You've checked the therapist's credentials, and you feel content with what you have learned. Your next step is to call the therapist and make an appointment for your initial interview and hope your chosen therapist has available time.

You might want to think of this step as akin to going on a (symbolic *only*) "first date." Like a date, when you set this first appointment you will call, ask a few questions, listen to the responses, get a sense of the person on the other end of the line and, based upon your conscious feelings and intuition, you will say yes or no to setting up an appointment. The theme here is to never detach from your perceptions. Then you will use the first appointment to see how you feel and to see if there is a workable "chemistry" between the two of you. If there is, you can make a second appointment. If not, you will explain your decision and gracefully part ways with no hard feelings.

That first phone call and first appointment might go better, however, if you have a list of questions to ask to help you determine whether this therapist is a good "fit." This chapter offers a few key questions to ask, as well as some essential warning signs to listen for when making your initial call to a potential psychotherapist.

The Initial Call: What to Ask

Some of you may already know this—if so, skip to the next chapter—but some will not: unless you are calling for an appointment at a clinic, hospital or university, you will mostly likely speak directly to the psychotherapist (or, since most of us don't have assistants, be asked to leave a voicemail message). If by chance you do reach a receptionist, ask to speak to the therapist in person. One of the most critical things to evaluate is whether you feel any kind of connection with the therapist and get the feeling that he/ she is someone who can help you. Even if you have to call back later, or leave a voicemail asking for a time to call back, make it a priority to speak directly to the therapist.

(As a former Ethics Committee member, I must stress again that before making your call, check the websites of the various professional boards and state organizations for any complaints filed against this particular therapist. There is no need to take a risk when there are many uncompromised therapists available from which to select.)

Since you might be feeling a bit anxious, have the following list of questions in front of you so you will remember the important questions to ask. When you reach the practitioner on the phone, introduce yourself and let them know how you got their name (through personal referral, a clinic, another clinician, etc.). This will give the therapist a context and information about you.

Then you should ask these questions at a minimum.

- *"Do you treat _____ (your particular issue)?"*
Or you can say something like, "I'm looking for a therapist who can help me with _____," and then describe your situation in a few clear sentences. Save the details of your situation for your first session unless asked. Make the assumption that they are asking you for a foreshortened version. For now, you want to present the therapist with an brief overview of the kind of help you are seeking, and whether he feels competent and has experience in that area.

- *"Do you have any openings?"* or *"Are you taking new patients?"*
Many good therapists are completely booked and not accepting new patients. If this is the case with this therapist, ask him/her for a referral to another practitioner, ask them if they have a waiting list, or move on to one of the other therapists on your list.

- *"How often do you typically see the patients you treat?"*
Weekly? More than once a week? Be prepared for the therapist to say, "That depends on what is needed." Most good therapists will want to get to know a patient and what their challenges are before recommending a particular number of sessions per week.

- *"What do you charge for a session?"*
  You want to know what their basic fees are. Most psychotherapists charge by the hour, and they schedule one-hour
  (actually 45 or 50 minutes) sessions with their patients.

- *"Do you take (your particular health insurance), if any?"*
  Some therapists will accept certain insurance plans but not
  other plans. If you have a PPO plan, they may require you
  to pay their fee and then submit the invoice for reimbursement. Many therapists have stopped accepting insurance
  at all because of the hassle of processing claims. If they
  don't accept any insurance and if their fees are beyond your
  budget, you can ask if they offer a payment plan or sliding
  fee scale. Don't hesitate to ask for names of other therapists
  they would recommend that might accept your particular
  insurance or have fees more suited to your budget.

- *"Can you tell me a little about your background?"*
  Depending on where you got the name of the therapist
  (a personal referral from a friend, a recommendation from
  your physician, or a name you received from a hospital,
  university, or clinic), you also may want to ask a few questions about the therapist's background and qualifications.
  Because it is relatively easy to find background information
  about therapists online—through the American Psychological Association or other professional organizations, for
  example—it may not be necessary to pursue this information over the telephone.

These questions should take no more than five to ten minutes
for the therapist to answer. If after this initial exchange you feel

satisfied and listened to, I suggest that you make an appointment to further explore the therapeutic relationship. Most experienced psychotherapists prefer face-to-face encounters rather than lengthy phone conversations. Generally a well-trained clinician's goal is to explore your concerns in the privacy of their office so they can be ready and able to offer support and empathy should painful material emerge, as it sometimes does. And remember, the initial phone call is not a free therapy session, so please don't expect the therapist to make treatment recommendations or suggestions.

Like other medical professionals, therapists are not magicians; they need upfront and personal contact with you to be able to help you. If you had a skin condition, for instance, and called a dermatologist, you might describe your general symptoms (an itchy, scaly patch on your arm), but any reputable doctor who didn't know you already would insist on seeing you in person before offering a diagnosis or a valid treatment plan. The same thing is doubly true with psychotherapy. Depending on your ability to openly discuss your situation, it may even take two, three, or more sessions before a therapist knows enough about you your history, your personality, or your distress before he or she can offer a treatment plan. I personally prefer to see someone three times before I agree to accept him or her as a patient. This gives the patient a greater sense of who I am and how I work, and me a greater sense of whether I am the best therapist for this individual.

If you have the need to describe all of your symptoms on the phone, it is often a sign of great anxiety, or an indication that your need for an appointment is more urgent than you realize. It may prompt the therapist to make time available sooner rather than later. If this is the case, typically a therapist at the end of the initial phone call might say, "It sounds like you've got a lot going on, would you like to make an appointment?" And, assuming that this is someone with whom you feel at ease, it will be worth your time and money to schedule a session.

Some therapists who work in clinical settings (like a hospital or university) may have an online scheduling system that you can use to make an appointment. However, when you contact a therapist for the first time, I recommend that you call first and ask to speak to him or her on the phone. That phone call can give you a great deal of information, and not just in terms of fees, schedule, approach, and so on. Listen carefully (see below) and use your intuition to know if this is the therapist you wish to see—or not.

What to Listen For

When you first speak with a therapist, you may, in just a few minutes, get a "hit" on whether you feel comfortable enough to want to establish a therapeutic relationship. Unless you like what you hear, don't feel pressured to make an appointment. Use your intuition—your "spidey sense." Here are a few important "clues" to consider:

- Do you feel relatively secure/in tune with this person on the phone?

- Does the therapist seem to have time for your questions, or does she seem abrupt? If he is rushed, is there an explanation? Perhaps he is between sessions and wanting to just connect before making an appointment to talk later.

- Does he respond clearly to your questions about fees, scheduling, expectations, etc.?

- Does the therapist "promise" results in a particular number of sessions? If so, *run*—every patient is different, and a reputable therapist needs to get to know you before she can determine the course of your therapy.

- Does the therapist talk to you in a way that makes you feel comfortable? Respected? I believe that therapists should talk to their patients as equals, not with an attitude of superiority, i.e., "I'm the big, important doctor who is going to cure you." You want to have a conversation with someone who listens attentively to your concerns—someone with special knowledge, but not someone who asserts her authority.

- Most importantly, do you feel that this particular therapist cares about you and understands what you're saying? Do you speak the same language? You want a therapist that will challenge you and help you face whatever barrier stands in the way of reaching your goals. You also want to feel that the therapist cares about you and wants to help you resolve your particular issue—and you can probably get a sense of that even in the first phone contact.

Remember, the decision to proceed with this particular individual is yours. If you are not at ease, trust your intuition and end the conversation politely. Conversely, if you have the sense that you want to see this therapist, don't hesitate to make that first appointment.

What's Happening on the Other End of the Line

While you're talking and trying to get a sense of the interaction with the therapist, the therapist is listening to you and trying to determine whether or not he/she can be of help to you. Every good therapist limits the hours of their clinical work, and many become expert and knowledgeable in a limited number of conditions. Trustworthy clinicians want to make sure that they are the best fit for you and your particular concerns.

Responsible therapists are clear regarding their rates, whether they accept insurance, or if they accept your particular plan. If their rates are too high, or they don't accept your insurance and you ask them for a referral, they should ask questions such as, "Do you prefer to see a man or a woman?" "Do you have any time limitations?" and "What fee range would be acceptable for you if you have to cover the cost of therapy out of pocket?"

Many people are discouraged by the cost of therapy, especially since many therapists recommend seeing patients once a week or more, for an indeterminate duration of time. The question you must consider is, "Is it worth the money and time expended to get the relief I want?" Would you prefer to see someone who accepts your insurance (or is within your HMO) even if you don't feel quite comfortable with that individual? Paying for the best therapist for you may require an additional financial commitment on your part, but if that therapist provides clarity and perspective to your thinking, it may be well worth the additional expense and time.

The First Appointment

In 1998, security expert Gavin de Becker published *The Gift of Fear*. In it, he wrote about the importance of learning to trust your instincts. We all have a sense of normalcy and can, by and large, determine when something is secure and when something is amiss. So, when you enter the therapist's office, be acutely aware of your instincts, to listen carefully for any warning signs or signals from your intuition telling you about the environment as well as the individual sitting in the therapist's chair.

Use every sense available to you. What do you see in their office? What is the underlying tone of the therapist's voice? What are the odors in the office? There are environments that welcome you with an immediate sense of reassurance or calm—or not. Does this office feel healing, holding, and supportive? Or are words coming to mind, like: "She sounds distracted and looks bored." "This place is a dump, there are papers strewn all over, it looks disorganized and chaotic." "I think I smell alcohol coming from the therapist." "Will this environment distract me from concentrating on my own experience, or not be therapeutic for me?"

You already have some sense about the therapist from your initial phone conversation, but when you meet him or her in person you will gain additional information. Do you get the same impression of the therapist as you did on the telephone? Allowing for the anxiety of a first or even several session(s) in their presence, are you at ease? Do you feel welcomed but not smothered or held at a distance?

The first appointment will consist of the therapist listening and also asking some questions and you responding to them. As a rule, the psychotherapist will ask you to tell them what brought you to therapy in more detail than you did over the phone. Be as clear as possible about the reasons you are seeking help and what, to the best of your understanding, are your particular issues. Competent therapists ask questions to help them (and you) clarify your problems. As they do this, they will observe you and your reactions, and gain a greater sense of your issues based upon their expertise in the area. They may ask questions that help you to look at your problems from a different vantage point, or to clarify issues for themselves.

The therapist may or may not say a much during this first hour, but regardless of how much or little they speak, your task is to listen to what's being said, pay attention to what you feel, and observe the therapist's attitude, posture, attentiveness, and behavior during the entire session. Here are a few of the qualities you should look for.

- Are they attentive? Do you feel listened to? Are they demonstrating concern? The best practitioners have a kind heart and an abundance of empathy. They can also be challenging—not in a hurtful way, but in order to get beneath the surface. You want a therapist who understands your experience, your distress, and who is able to help you make sense of it. The best therapists that I have been to and know also have a good sense of humor.

- At the same time, they must be able to be objective about your issues while still being empathic. Good therapists can look at your issues dispassionately and objectively, but not *so* dispassionately and objectively that they appear aloof and judging. And they are not so empathic that they are unable to express the difficult words and impressions that therapists may sometimes have to say.

- Does the therapist ask questions that you have never asked yourself, questions that encourage you to open your mind to new understanding?

- Does the therapist challenge you? You don't want someone who is going to buy into your story, family history, or beliefs. Instead, you want someone who can confront your self-indulgences, your distortions, or your pathologic behavior—someone who is unafraid to call you on your "stuff." Several of my patients have said this or something similar, "You don't buy my bullsh*t."

- Bottom line, you should feel this therapist has experience, professionalism, maturity, good common sense, a good heart, empathy, and a commitment to advancing and enhancing your progress.

At the end of the beginning session, therapists typically take a few minutes to ask how you feel about the time you've spent together, and whether you have any questions. Don't be afraid to ask anything that comes to mind so you can make an informed choice. You may want to ask about the therapist's qualifications and training (if you haven't done so already on the phone). You might want to know if the therapist has ever been in therapy. This is a somewhat sensitive question for some, but I believe that a therapist must go through not "just" a therapeutic experience, but also a long-term, in-depth psychotherapy or psychoanalysis. This provides both a deeper self-understanding and the lived experience of what a patient feels. No one can teach what they have not lived and lived deeply.

The First Appointment: Warning Signs

As you engage with the therapist and they ask their questions, you should continue to pay attention to your feelings—your "gut," if you will—about what comes up, positive or negative. In particular, you should look for these warning signs.

- Is the therapist defensive when you ask a question? Or alternatively, is the therapist too self-revealing, telling you more than you wanted to know? There is a happy medium. Often the questions you ask have significance, and for that reason, the therapist may sometimes delay answering. If he does not have the capacity to be reasonably and appropriately open about himself, you might feel unable to trust him, or the process. I don't mean they are there to tell you "their story." In fact, this is your time, and your session should be devoted to you. Yet if you feel the therapist is too guarded or defensive, or too self-revealing, most likely he is not the right psychotherapist for you.

- Is there any sense that the therapist is going to take advantage of you—financially, emotionally, sexually, or otherwise?

- An effective therapist will ask questions that may make you look at uncomfortable issues or truths about your behavior, but please understand that there is a difference between that reasonable discomfort and the sensation that the therapist is asking inappropriate questions, especially in the first meeting. It is important that a relationship of trust is established first before embarking on the deep questions that might ensue later in the treatment. If you feel that the therapist is overstepping boundaries, trust yourself and walk.

From the Therapist's Side

At the same time you are evaluating the therapist, she will be evaluating you as a potential patient to determine if the two of you are a good enough fit. An experienced therapist will wonder if her therapeutic approach and personal style will achieve the positive therapeutic outcome desired. She will assess your response to her questions and consider your defensiveness or openness. In other words, she wants to know if your style of communicating meshes with hers. She hopefully will be asking herself if her style is too confrontational, or not challenging enough for you.

Some patients, for example, find my approach intimidating because I am direct and unwilling to *not* discuss the "elephant(s) in the room." I am not interested in wasting anyone's time and precious resources if my style feels too challenging. Indeed, many patients prefer my approach *because* they don't trust what they experience as an overly supportive, approach where little growth takes place.

A thoughtful therapist asks herself questions like, "Am I the best therapist to work with this person? Do I respect him? Can I empathize with him rather than be judgmental? Will I learn to care about him? Do I truly care about his stated goals and values and not in any way impose mine?"

Some of my patients have been known to say, "It sometimes feels as if you want more for my life than I think is possible." It is often true that people are unable to muster the hope required to change, and a caring competent therapist believing more in them than they do themselves (in that moment) is a positive reaction. If the ultimate answer is yes and you believe the therapist and the environment are suitable for therapeutic success, then this is probably the therapist for you.

After the First Appointment

After the first visit, ask yourself if you know more about yourself and what's going on than you did before entering the therapist's office. If so, you should schedule at least two more sessions to make certain this is what I call a "good enough" fit. Nothing is perfect. A therapeutic relationship is similar to any other relationship: while the first appointment tells you a lot, you usually need to have a few more appointments before you make any kind of commitment. As I mentioned earlier, I prefer to see patients at least three times before agreeing to begin treatment. I want to make sure I can help them with the issues they are facing, and to do that I need a greater sense of what and how they are dealing with their problems than I can get in one meeting. I also want to be confident that the patient experiences my way of being with them as beneficial—not too severe, not too comfy, but just right. Think of the Goldilocks story: you are looking for a good enough fit.

Assuming the therapist accepts you as a patient, he will usually propose a time for your next appointment and a therapy schedule: once a week, twice a week, sometimes even more depending on the type of therapist you have chosen and the problems you confront. After two or three sessions, you both can evaluate your progress. In the next chapter we will cover what to expect from the therapeutic relationship over time, how you should feel if it's working, and what to do if therapy isn't producing the results you want.

7

WHAT TO EXPECT IN THE THERAPEUTIC RELATIONSHIP

"Find a place inside where there's joy,
and the joy will burn out the pain."

JOSEPH CAMPBELL

A therapeutic relationship is like any other—it needs to be harmonious for both parties if it's going to accomplish the therapeutic goal. As the patient, you need to feel a connection and a sense of trust in order for the relationship to work. If you have had trouble trusting in the past, chances are that you will confront the same problem in therapy. Hopefully, one of your goals will be to change that.

Remember, therapy is an exploration and a journey, and the relationship with your therapist will unfold over several sessions. One of the reasons I recommend that people schedule a minimum of three sessions with a psychotherapist before committing to a long-term therapy plan is that within three sessions you both should have a good idea of whether this therapeutic relationship will work or not. Have you learned something that has given you some relief or hope, or even greater understanding? Have you garnered an insight that has helped you understand something previously unknown? At the very least, you should have a conviction—an abiding perception—that this therapist can help you.

After the first three sessions, it is plausible for you to ask the therapist for his or her thoughts or expectations regarding your treatment. This is the time for you to ask questions about the frequency of sessions, the expected length of the treatment, and so forth. No reputable psychotherapist can tell you that within so many sessions you will feel X, or within a year such-and-such X will happen. Each patient is different, and progress depends on the individual, the issues, and the self-awareness he or she brings to the table. If someone stubbornly resists another perspective— having to "be the one who knows," for example—I am confident that this kind of treatment will take longer than someone who is less defensive and more eager or capable of doing the work to learn and evolve. Be willing to have a frank discussion with the therapist to get an idea of how they see your therapy progressing and their recommendations for scheduling, based on what they've learned about you and about your issues.

Here are some significant qualities that make for a good therapeutic relationship.

You can respect the therapist and feel you can learn from her.

Do you admire and see your therapist as a potential role model? Do you believe this person has something to teach you? Is this therapist several steps ahead of you, assisting you in perceiving things in a new light? Remember, therapy is not just designed to deal with your emotions or to help you process and mourn the past mistakes or failures. Therapy should foster finding a pathway out of the circumstances that have thwarted your happiness and success.

You don't need a babysitter and a hand-holder. Instead, you want someone who empathizes *and* helps you move forward.

A good therapist is not just someone with whom to cry. Of course, you want your therapist to listen to your emotions with compassion and empathy. But remember, your therapist is not your best friend, boyfriend or girlfriend, mother or father. His job is not just to console you, although at times he may do that. If, however, the only thing your therapist says is, "I can imagine how upsetting that is, and I'm so sorry for those losses in your life," it will not lead to enlightenment and additional understanding. To talk with someone who is empathic can certainly make you feel better in the moment. But you don't want (again) a "kiss the boo-boo" therapist, because the only thing you will walk away with is, "I feel better for the moment, but I'm still the same place with the same hurdles to jump over."

Your therapist should certainly sit with you through your sadness and tears, but her primary responsibility is to shed light on what created this unproductive situation and then help you to reframe it so that you can move on. After all the compassion, her next questions might be, "What can we learn about this? Where are the lessons in what's happened? What are your next steps? How can we understand this so that you don't continue to repeat the same situation over and over again? And if you, do what's in it for you? What reward might you be getting that is causing you to repeat this behavior? Are you unknowingly seeking attention you feel you wouldn't otherwise receive? Or, might you be confusing sympathy for love?" You need a therapist who will engage with you and encourage you see things in a different way.

You want a therapist who is able to be objective, one who questions your assumptions and can see your blind spots.

Good therapists must be objective when they look at your situation, and part of their job is to get you to be more objective, as well. They do this in several ways. First, they will look for what's holding you back, your past roadblocks: what beliefs, memories, or excuses you have used that keep you from being your "ideal" self. From their objective vantage point, they will observe and comment upon your behavior, your resistance, the thinking that underlies the behavior that keeps you running in place.

Second, they will question your assumptions and your beliefs. As they listen to you, they may hear things that don't make sense—distortions like the way you continue to believe that your brother was a good big brother who always protected you in spite of the fact that he tormented you as soon as your parents left the room. Effective therapists pose questions that illuminate what can sometimes feel like the darker, hidden feelings and conflicts, things that you have resisted knowing. We often begin by resisting "knowing" because we fear to face the truth. We are afraid we won't be able to maintain certain relationships or tolerate the pain. Trust me, it is more painful to continue to live with the deceit and distortions than to endure the very pain that is responsible for our suffering. A good therapist will help connect the dots that have somehow eluded you, and in so doing, uncover the mistaken beliefs that have wounded your psyche and impeded your growth.

There may be a time that you will leave a session feeling a

bit discombobulated and resisting an interpretation that your therapist offered. After reflecting upon the exchange, you may hear yourself saying, "I never thought of it that way," or, "I just didn't want to see it in that way." And perhaps the next day, you might look forward to your session and proudly proclaim, "I really thought about what we were talking about and, in thinking it over, I believe we're onto something." Then you and your therapist will know that you're on the right track to something meaningful.

You want a therapist who will challenge your thinking.

Some of the best therapists are those who are not afraid to confront their patients with difficult interpretations about their past history and actions, their current behavior, etc. An experienced therapist will question your behavior. They may ask questions like: "What's going on?" Or, "I have a hunch what you're doing feels familiar. How can we understand this?"

You want a therapist to challenge the expectations you have for yourself, to challenge what you believe about your past, or about what is possible or you hope for the future. While this will not always be warm and comfortable and you may squirm a bit, it is an essential but necessary step in order to nudge you out of the rut that brought you to treatment in the first place. A first-rate therapist can be an "adjunct mind" to assist you to think (and feel) your way out of where you are now—stuck and repeating old patterns—so you can arrive at your goal.

You should feel that the therapist is "in it to win it" for you— and vice versa.

I believe that therapists are often "temporary backbones" for their patients. "You don't believe change is possible? Lean on me, because I believe that with a little support for a little while, it is doable for you." You should have the sense that if you falter along the way, your therapist is there for you to lean on, to help you pick yourself up and dust yourself off. Equally important, you should feel that your therapist can envisage more for you than you can for yourself, and they are committed to your progress and goals.

Patients have said to me, "I'm not sure if this is my goal or your goal." Of course I want to hear what they feel and think, but chances are that I have heard their dreams for the future over and over, and yet they remain only dreams. Often, my expressed goal is one they have expressed and *could* achieve—but for the fear of changing. The proverb "Better the devil you know than the angel you don't" is an accurate reflection of this resistance to change. You've lived this way a long time and know what it feels like and how to survive. But changing? That's downright scary and hard.

For my *Challenge Your Thinking* podcast I interview people who achieve amazing feats, and they too are scared. It's frightening to go beyond what we imagine and know. Therapists are not about creating goals for you, but we *are* about recognizing strengths and talents you have displayed but are unaware of. You have hired your therapist to do just that: to work hard to help you see the world through a more realistic lens, one without the roadblocks that encumbered you in the past.

In order to be successful, you must be willing to risk change, and be completely honest with yourself. This isn't always easy. Being curious rather than resistant about the therapist's insights will leave you more open to change. You need to be ready to face the truth of your past, mourn the pain, and take responsibility (not blame) for your part (where appropriate) in the issues you are confronting. And whatever your issues, you need to be committed to addressing them proactively for your treatment to flourish.

Be willing to process things with a goal to ultimately move forward.

For many people, part of the therapeutic process is dealing with unresolved issues, unproductive emotions, or unprocessed trauma. The goal of therapy is to process these feelings and issues to come to a new understanding, and ultimately *to get on with your life*. In the beginning, your achievement will feel like "baby steps," but if you're willing to do what it takes (mourn your losses, feel your feelings, take some risks, change your behavior, look at your own behavior) you will, little by little, get to the next level of maturity and sound mental health. You can grieve the past and at the same time capture something new and different that you want to create in your life. In fact, having a clear picture of a better future is one of the most important goals and results of successful therapy.

Most of us have experienced trauma: losing a loved one, experiencing a car crash, child abuse, physical or emotional abuse. What we *do* with the trauma is what will affect the outcome. Do we grieve the tragedy for the remainder of our lives rather than doing the work of mourning and eventually making an accommodation to it and living the best we can? Please understand, many of these issues take time, tears, and struggle. But we do have a choice to acknowledge the trauma and somehow find the strength and resilience to move forward. And in doing so, we become stronger.

I am a firm believer in what Michaela Haas, Ph.D., author of *Bouncing Forward*, calls "post-traumatic growth." After trauma, some people refuse to be victims and, as a result, they discover the strength and resilience they never knew they had. For example, consider Candace Lightner, who lost a child to a car crash caused by a drunk driver and went on to found MADD, Mothers Against Drunk Driving. She turned one of her life's most difficult challenges to the benefit of others by saving hundreds of thousands of lives.

Whatever your trauma or past challenges, you must be willing to face them, deal with them, and hopefully move past them. Good therapists will encourage you to give up being a victim for the rest of your life. Their goal is to help you move past your past and to create a better present and future for yourself. And you must be an active participant in that process.

As Your Therapy Progresses

As your sessions accrue, you should feel that you comprehend more about the issues that brought you to therapy. This is not to say that you won't resist change. Likely, you will. Change is one of the hardest things to commit to in life. Ask yourself several questions: Do you see things more clearly? Have you learned things about yourself? Are you more curious about the way you think? Are you less fearful about what's inside? Having a trusted therapist on the path to health and healing, someone to guide you in the direction toward emotional wisdom and good mental health, is not only uplifting but also necessary. From there, "progress" will depend on you and your therapist. However, some of the things you might notice are:

You feel relieved. The first feeling my patients often express is one of relief. They feel like they can take a deep breath again; they begin to experience more "psychic space" and feel more energetic. It is vital to address the stumbling blocks of your life with someone who provides an empathetic, judicious, yet objective perspective.

You start asking better questions about your emotions and actions. Part of the goal of therapy is to start questioning yourself—not in a self-doubting or blaming/shameful way, but from the vantage point of becoming more and more inquisitive about yourself, your internal life, your decisions and the reason for making them. Instead of asking questions like, "What's wrong with me?" you ask, "What do I think?" "How do I feel?" "What do I want?" "What matters to me?" and, "Is this decision a repetition of those I've made in the past that haven't worked?" In the course of treatment, many people learn to question themselves in ways that will reflect their growing sense of self-esteem and the courage to look honestly at themselves. In other words, no blame, no guilt.

You learn better life skills, such as being at ease with solitude, or taking on challenging projects at work or in your personal life. Hopefully, you have learned to self-soothe in sustainable ways without relying on psychological crutches like food, alcohol, the internet, or porn (to name a few). For some, this can take years. Hopefully, you have achieved abilities and emotional proficiencies that provide for healthier life choices.

You have a sense that you are progressing in the right direction. Yes, there may (and probably will) be setbacks and frustrations along the way. You might even feel worse at times during therapy because you are confronting painful memories, powerful emotions, and destructive behaviors you have long ignored. But with an effectual therapist who is willing to confront while emotionally (not literally) "holding" you and your vision of what is most beneficial, those anxieties should diminish, and you should have the sense that life is progressing in a constructive and positive direction.

What to Do If It's Not Working

On one hand, if you are attending sessions and you feel things are not progressing, then it may be time to raise your concerns with the therapist. Maybe expressing your previously hidden emotions and issues in therapy has left you feeling somewhat improved for reason of the catharsis—but it's not lasting. Or perhaps after many sessions over a period of time you feel stymied because you feel your therapist is mostly "just listening" with little or no interaction. Or maybe, despite therapy, you are still plagued with what feels like the status quo that brought you to therapy in the first place.

If this is so, it's time to have a frank discussion with your therapist and to communicate these concerns. It is in your therapist's best interests, as well as your own, for you to have a positive therapeutic experience, and that includes getting results. A therapist must be open to listening to you explore your expectations. They may be able to clarify your concerns so that you will feel optimistic about continuing as their patient. Or you may both decide that it would be better for you to see a different therapist. Remember, if the relationship is not working, it's not necessarily the fault of either of you. It's just possible that you weren't a good enough fit to begin with, and it took some sessions to come to that conclusion.

However, there are some specific "red flags" to watch out for during your treatment.

Unprofessional conduct. Does your therapist talk about other patients, or share any information about them with you? That's a big red flag. Just as your treatment is strictly confidential and private, so should the treatment of their other patients be restricted to the therapy room.

Charging you more than they said they would. If you are paying with insurance, there may be some exchange of information with the insurance company about payment, but the therapist should have previously told you what the fee for each session is, and that should not change without discussing it with you.

Lack of boundaries. Let's say in the course of your session you mention that you plan to put your house up for sale, and the therapist says, "Oh, I know a really great realtor—she's my cousin. Would you like her number?" Big problem... even something as innocent sounding as recommending a family member to you for a service can muddy the waters of the therapist/patient relationship. You need to feel that the therapist is there completely for your benefit, and only yours. Any referral given to you by your therapist should have no secondary gain for them.

It's important for your therapist to maintain the proper boundaries, and it's also important for you to understand why it might be hard for you to do the same. (Sexual abuse and incest survivors in particular have difficulty understanding this because the proper boundaries were not respected or held for them.) No matter what the situation, it is important for you and your therapist to talk about it and come to a greater understanding. There are *never* valid reasons to violate boundaries unless patients are about to harm themselves or others. Boundaries are there to protect you, and they are put in place for the protection of both the therapist and the patient. Ultimately, it is your therapist's responsibility and duty to keep the relationship strictly professional.

Some patients may become attracted to their therapist. At times that is inevitable; it is called transference. However, just like a parent, it is the therapist's responsibility to only listen to your feelings of attraction and to help you understand what you may be feeling. If you ever sense that your therapist might be receptive to and encouraging your "transference" feeling, *run*. In *no* world is it permissible for patients to have a romantic relationship with their therapist. If there is any kind of attraction that both parties would like to pursue (and I am against this), it is the therapist's responsibility to end the therapeutic relationship immediately, seek consultation, and refer the patient to another therapist. You can check with your local Board or Ethics Committee to confirm that relationships between therapists and patients are never warranted or recommended. In fact, they are an abuse of power.

It is *never* okay for a therapist and patient to date or to become sexually involved. Professional boards consider that behavior a violation of their ethical codes. Therapists have a responsibility to serve the best interests of their patients first, last, and *always*, and getting involved romantically is *never* serving the patients' best interest.

Whatever the reason you feel that your treatment, or this therapist, is unsatisfactory and going no place, talk to your therapist first but don't hesitate to end the treatment and look for someone else. Ending treatment with your therapist can be painful and difficult. However, the only way you can find the *right* therapist is to be willing to leave the wrong one—cleanly, clearly, and as quickly as possible. Try to think of it as a sign of growth and strength.

Of course, my hope is that by reading this book and following my suggestions you will be able to make the right choice from the get-go. Most therapists are eager to help you, and they want you to succeed in eliminating the barriers that have impeded your happiness and success. They want you to do well and eventually walk out of their office feeling that you will go on to create the life you desire, that you are strong and have the emotional tools to handle the challenges most people face. They want you to develop a self that is authentic—one that reflects your "true self" rather than one that serves to please others. They will miss you when you leave, but they will be proud of the progress you have made through your commitment and honored that you chose to do the work with them.

8

CONCLUSION:
AT THE CROSSROADS OF HEALTH

*"When it comes to personal happiness there is a lot
that we as individuals can do."*

THE DALAI LAMA

Congratulations. You are standing at the crossroads, and you are ready to take your first steps on the path to greater health and contentment. I wrote this book to give you the information you need to take those steps with greater confidence, to find the therapist that's right for you—hopefully in your first attempt—who will best suit your needs and will be with you on your journey.

No therapist can do the work for you; that's your job. But we *can* and want to be at your side, encouraging you, pointing you in the right direction and helping you to keep moving even when the going gets tough. I can't guarantee that therapy will turn your life from "a trainwreck" into "nirvana." No therapist can make that promise. But if you follow the steps in this book and use them to choose a "good enough" therapist as your guide, I believe that you will be on the path to a happier, more successful, healthier, more meaningful and authentic life.

I wish you all the best on your journey to health and a greater sense of well-being. And, I would be honored if you would consider letting me know how you're doing.

SUMMARY

11 TIPS TO FINDING THE RIGHT PSYCHOTHERAPIST FOR YOU

#1: There are different kinds of therapy and therapists. Find the one that's *right* for you.

#2: Your therapist can come from your local area—or not. Some skilled therapists work over the phone or via Skype. However, there is something of value in the face-to-face, in-person interaction of therapist and patient.

#3: While the two most common ways to pay for therapy is through health insurance and out-of-pocket, there are other, lower-cost options available through university graduate programs and psychotherapist training institutes.

#4: Choose the best sources for a referral to a therapist. They include: friends, family, and therapy training programs at local universities. Your primary care physician may or may not be a good referral source. However, use the internet only for the verification of your own research.

#5: The initial call with the therapist should tell you a lot. Do you feel safe and in attunement with the therapist on the phone? If so, make an appointment. Make sure to ask about the fee and whether or not the therapist accepts insurance up front so there are no surprises.

#6: Let your instincts be your guide in the first appointment and moving forward. Make sure you feel comfortable in the therapist's office and that nothing feels amiss.

#7: You want a therapist to challenge you, not "kiss the boo-boo and make it better." Therapy is designed to open your mind to new experiences and to explore your thoughts and emotions, and your therapist is your guide and partner in that process.

#8: Therapy may be a years-long process or a short-term program. Let it take the time required for success. Don't expect instant results, but *do* expect growth and progress along the way, and especially over time.

#9: Know your boundaries, and if your therapist crosses them (by proposing a relationship outside of therapy, for example) leave—and know that you have the option of reporting the therapist to their licensing board.

#10: Your progress will depend on staying the course and working hard to understand yourself. Your therapist is your therapeutic partner, but ultimately you need to be willing to address the issues in your life without blame or guilt.

#11: The way you know therapy is effective is that you feel better, less depressed or anxious, and/or able to get along better with friends and colleagues. Most importantly, you are able to see yourself more clearly, to take responsibility for both the positive and negative conditions of your life, and able to make corrections should you momentarily lose your balance. Find a good therapist to be your guide and you will find your way to authenticity, emotional maturity and psychological health.

For a free special report by Dr. Linda Tucker,
7 Tips to Moving Forward Faster in 7 Days:
How to Challenge Your Thinking and
Accelerate Your Healing in Just One Week,
please go to www.drlindatucker.com/7tips/
and enter your email.

ABOUT LINDA TUCKER,

PsyD, LCSW

With a combined depth of experience that spans 35 years, Dr. Linda Tucker helps many individuals and couples lead more fulfilling lives. Her successful private practice as a psychotherapist, couples therapist, psychoanalyst and "coaches' coach" in the San Francisco Bay Area for over 20 years emerged from 15 years as a counselor at various East Coast and Bay Area nonprofit organizations. She also has worked with many professionals at various stages of their careers to catapult them to partnerships, executive level positions, and philanthropy.

In addition to her clinical practice in downtown San Francisco, Dr. Tucker has instructed and supervised students at Bay Area colleges, universities and institutes. She was honored by many of her students and colleagues, who voted her "one of San Francisco's Best Psychologists."

Dr. Tucker has co-founded, developed, facilitated, and coordinated many nonprofit programs in the San Francisco Bay Area. She currently serves on the Advisory Board to Access Institute for Psychological Services, where she is the Past President of the Board of Directors and the former Board Development Chair. Access Institute is one of the premier Bay Area Post Doctoral training programs and delivers affordable psychological services for those without adequate insurance or the means to afford high-quality, longer-term treatment. Dr. Tucker also serves on the Advisory Board of WeSaveLives.org.

As an active member of numerous professional organizations and associations, Dr. Tucker dedicates numerous volunteer hours providing *pro bono* psychotherapy and consultation for various Bay Area nonprofits. Currently, she is on the volunteer roster to provide psychotherapy services for Giving an Hour, and The Coming Home Project. Both of these organizations provide therapeutic services for returning veterans and their families.

Dr. Tucker received a Masters in Clinical Social Work from the University of California at Berkeley, completed her post-master's psychodynamic training at the Psychotherapy Institute in Berkeley, and received her Doctorate in Psychoanalysis from the Psychoanalytic Institute of Northern California. Additionally, she has pursued couples therapy training and consultation with many prominent psychoanalysts and couples therapy theorists and researchers from around the world. Dr. Tucker's publications, papers, studies, and podcasts cover such topics as overcoming fear, roadblocks to success, relationships, living with integrity, sex abuse, body image, eating disorders, and people who use porn, strippers and/or cheating as a defense against intimacy.

With a Communications degree and as the former host of a radio program, Dr. Tucker also has created two documentary films and a Podcast. One of these films is about a psychoanalytic icon, Dr. Hedda Bolgar. Her award-winning, "What's Hot" and "Featured" iTunes *Challenge Your Thinking* podcast was created to inspire others to overcome fear and move forward in their lives and in their relationships.

Dr. Tucker grew up on the East Coast and did some of her initial psychological training in New York City. She currently resides in San Francisco.

For more information, please visit www.drlindatucker.com.

ABOUT THE

CHALLENGE YOUR THINKING PODCAST

In Dr. Linda Tucker's award-winning iTunes podcast, *Challenge Your Thinking*, she interviews *New York Times* bestselling authors, athletes, psychologists, researchers, entrepreneurs, and experts in many fields, including Amy Cuddy (*Presence*), Adam Grant (*Originals*), Simon Sinek (*Start with Why*), Gay Hendricks (*The Big Leap*), Candace Lightner (founder of MADD), and many more.

Guests like Jen Bricker (born without legs, she became a top aerialist and entertainer in Las Vegas), Trina Laughlin (a trauma therapist who faced trauma herself when she lost her son), Sudeep Balain (divorce launched him on a quest to find personal and spiritual growth), Beth French (who got out of a wheelchair to become the first swimmer to swim the channels of the seven continents in one year), Felicity Aston (the first and only woman/person to cross the South Pole alone), and Richard McCann (who found peace when he forgave his mother's murderer) have faced trauma, extreme challenges and difficult circumstances in their lives and businesses, and then used their experiences and failures to become better, stronger, wiser, and in the process have become inspirational to others.

Every week their stories inspire listeners to do more to overcome their own challenges and change their thinking. You too may find these people powerful examples that will help you overcome your own obstacles as you seek your own healing.

If you'd like to listen or learn more, please go to www.drlindatucker.com/podcast.

ACKNOWLEDGMENTS

This book would not be possible were it not for my patients and consultees; they inspire me almost every day to keep doing what I love.

Some of the mentors, psychologists and psychoanalysts who have contributed to my growth are listed here chronologically: Dennis Seale, Irving Solomon, PhD, Lillian Johnson, LCSW, Maureen Murphy, PhD, Shelley Alhanati, PhD, Robert Oelsner, MD, and Stanley Steinberg, MD. I mean it when I say that each and every one of these individuals has enriched my life and expanded my heart and ability to trust that when you reach out, someone will reach back.

My friendship with Amy Gentile, PhD, spans over forty years. We have shared many things in one another's life including our very first therapist. She was there at an important analytic crossroads in my life. I have many more dear friends who are too numerous to mention who all know they have my love and thanks.

Editors are invaluable and, as such, I consider myself fortunate to have a guide and mentor as experienced as Victoria St. George of Just Write Editorial and Literary Services. I consider her my guardian angel and have her to thank for holding my hand while taking my first steps as an author. A very special thanks goes out to Judy Robinett for being who she is and for sharing Vicki with me.

Kare Anderson (as did Judy) started out as a guest on my podcast. As an Emmy Award winning journalist, who has become a special force in my life, she gently pushed me to go way beyond my comfort zone. I always believed that I would write a book; Kare makes it possible to believe that this is only my first.

My psychoanalytic "left tackle" and dear friend, Barbara Artson, PhD, was invaluable in the process of writing this book. She has always had my back in the written word, as well as in the real world. Without her eyes, ears and editing talents I would not have felt as secure to reach this goal line.

Many people have catapulted me forward. I have mentioned several, but some deserve a special category of their own. They are: Tsipora Peskin, DSW, Glen Gabbard, MD, Kim Krompass, CPA, and Harvey Peskin, PhD. They each hold a very special place in my heart and psyche.

I was fortunate to know and have Dr. Hedda Bolgar, PhD, as my mentor and incredible friend. Her faith, love, and trust in me continue even without her physical presence. I will always miss you. The life you led was an inspiration to many and I will do it justice and fulfill the promises I made to you.

Without love, life isn't as sweet. My life partner is the one who believes in me (dare I say) almost more than I believe in myself, and our two boys make life more meaningful and fun.

Here is what I believe: The success of another is inspiration for another. And, all of these people have inspired me and continue to lift me up in one way or another.

I have deep gratitude for each and everyone listed here and several who are not.

Final note: This book was about finding the right psychotherapist; however, finding the right mentors in our lives can be equally important and inspiring.

BIBLIOGRAPHY

American Psychiatric Association. (2013). *Diagnostic and statistical manual of mental disorders, fifth edition.* Washington, DC: American Psychiatric Publishing.

Anxiety and Depression Association of America. (2016). Facts & statistics. Retrieved March 28, 2017 from the ADAA website: www.adaa.org/about-adaa/press-room/facts-statistics.

Campbell, Joseph & Moyers, Bill. (1988). The Power of Myth: Programs 1-6 (television series). PBS.

DSM-5 List of Mental Disorders. Retrieved March 28, 2017 from Psychology Charts website: www.psychologycharts.com/list-of-mental-disorders.html.

Haas, Michaela, PhD. (2015). *Bouncing forward: transforming bad breaks into breakthroughs.* New York: Enliven Books/Atria.

Mental health by the numbers. Retrieved March 28, 2017 from the NAMI website: www.nami.org/Learn-More/Mental-Health-By-the-Numbers.

National Alliance on Mental Illness. (2017). Mental health conditions. Retrieved March 28, 2017 from NAMI website: www.nami.org/Learn-More/Mental-Health-Conditions.

National Institute of Mental Health. (2017). Health topics. Retrieved March 28, 2017 from NIMH website: www.nimh.nih.gov/index. shtml.

U.S. Department of Health & Human Services. (2017). Mental health myths and facts. Retrieved March 28, 2017 from the HHS website: www.mentalhealth.gov/basics/myths-facts/.

Winnicott, D.W. (1953). Transitional objects and transitional phenomena—a study of the first not-me possession. *International Journal of Psycho-Analysis, 34,* 89-97.

NOTES

1 "Finding your bliss" is Joseph Campbell's elegant term for the pursuit of one's happiness. See Campbell, Joseph & Moyers, Bill. (1988). The Power of Myth: Programs 1-6 (television series). PBS.

2 Winnicott, D.W. (1953). Transitional objects and transitional phenomena—a study of the first not-me possession. *International Journal of Psycho-Analysis, 34*, 89-97.

3 The information on common mental health conditions is drawn from these resources:
American Psychiatric Association. (2013). *Diagnostic and statistical manual of mental disorders, fifth edition.* American Psychiatric Publishing, Washington, DC.
National Institute of Mental Health. (2017). Health topics. Retrieved March 28, 2017 from NIMH website: www.nimh.nih.gov/index.shtml.
National Alliance on Mental Illness. (2017). Mental health conditions. Retrieved March 28, 2017 from NAMI website: www.nami.org/Learn-More/Mental-Health-Conditions.
DSM-5 List of Mental Disorders. Retrieved March 28, 2017 from

Psychology Charts website: www.psychologycharts.com/list-of-mental-disorders.html.

4   The sources for these statistics are as follows: National Alliance on Mental Illness. (2016). Mental health by the numbers. Retrieved March 28, 2017 from the NAMI website: www.nami.org/Learn-More/Mental-Health-By-the-Numbers.

Anxiety and Depression Association of America. (2016). Facts & statistics. Retrieved March 28, 2017 from the ADAA website: www.adaa.org/about-adaa/press-room/facts-statistics.

U.S. Department of Health & Human Services. (2017). Mental health myths and facts. Retrieved March 28, 2017 from the HHS website: www.mentalhealth.gov/basics/myths-facts/.

www.ingramcontent.com/pod-product-compliance
Lightning Source LLC
Chambersburg PA
CBHW022339280326
41934CB00006B/697